HEALTH LIBRARY

FIRST
AID

FIRST
AID

© 2006 Ars Medica, Grupo Ars XXI, Barcelona, Spain
© 2006 Rebo Publishers

Concept and project management: Jordi Vigué
Editing of original version: Myriam Cañas
Correction: Ramon Aymerich
Medical consultant: Dr. Gonçal Folch
Photography: Archivo Fotográfico Gorg Blanc, Capsa Màgica Studio
Illustrations: Ana Journade, Roger Tallada, David Navarrot, Daniel Martínez
Arrangement of images: Rosa Rigau
Graphic Design: Celia Valero
Editorial coordination: Miquel Ridola

Layout: AdAm Studio, Prague, The Czech Republic
Typesetting and pre-press services: AdAm Studio, Prague, The Czech Republic
Translation: David Stow for First Edition Translations Ltd, Cambridge, UK
Editing: David Price for First Edition Translations Ltd, Cambridge, UK
Proofreading: Sarah Dunham

ISBN 13: 978-90-366-1908-0
ISBN 10: 90-366-1908-4

C O N T E N T S

ACCIDENT PREVENTION

ASSISTANCE TECHNIQUES

EMERGENCIES

Why is first aid important?

It has been proven that in an emergency, the first actions taken are crucial to the fate of the injured person. When professional help arrives, every attempt to treat the victim is made, but, the people present when a medical emergency occurs are those who have to take action first. Herein, therefore, lies the importance of first aid.

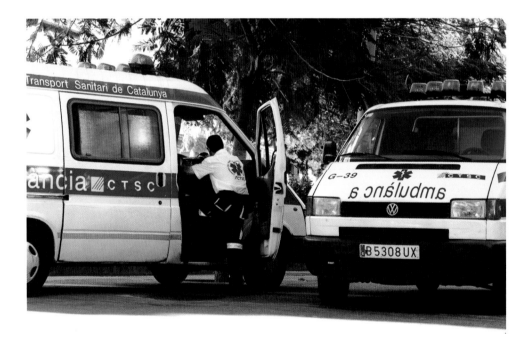

◼ Objectives of first aid

- Preserving life
- Reducing to a minimum the possible risk of injuries or later negative conse quences of the accident
- Avoiding later complications, either physical or psychological
- Aiding recovery
- Ensuring the transfer of the casualty to a medical center

When practicing first aid, it is advisable to follow a logical sequence known by the abbreviation PAA. These are the initials of the three actions that must be taken when attending to a person who has suffered an accident: Protect, Alert, and Assist.

What is first aid?

First aid is the immediate, appropriate and provisional care given to people before they are able to receive attention at a medical center.

By first aid we mean those measures and actions taken by a helper at the site of an accident with equipment that is often improvised until the arrival of specialized personnel. First aid does not consist of medical treatment, but rather emergency care aimed at reducing the effects of the injuries and stabilizing the condition of the victim. It is the latter that makes first aid so important. The general condition and later recovery of the casualty to a large extent depend upon these first actions taken.

Protect

It is fundamental, before taking any action, to consider the surroundings, so as to identify risks that might affect either the individual needing help, or others. The measures to be taken depend on where the accident has occurred, although in general they are the following:

- Put on protective gloves in case of wounds.
- Place warning signs at the site of the accident, if it took place on a road.
- Disconnect the electricity and the gas, if, for example the accident involves electrocution.

Alert

You will need to call for medical assistance, by phoning the emergency services' number. So it is useful to keep a list of the most important emergency telephone numbers: physician, ambulance, fire brigade, police, etc., in a place that is highly visible, well known and accessible to everyone (at home in the first aid kit and when traveling, with your most important documents).

Give precise information when reporting an accident

- The name of who is calling

- The number you are calling from

- The exact location of the accident. As many details as possible should be given

- The number of people involved

- Try to explain how the accident occurred

- The type of injuries or symptoms of the casualty

- Whether the victim has any special characteristics (an elderly • person, a baby, a pregnant woman, a physical or mental disability, etc.)

- The person calling should be the last to hang up, in case the emergency services need more information

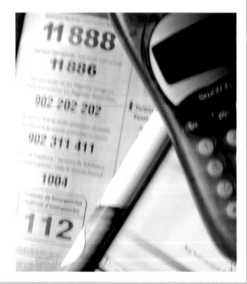

**Never move a sick or injured person if
there is any possibility of a spinal injury.
If the person has severe pain in the neck or spine,
a tingling sensation or loss of feeling in their
limbs, he should not be moved.**

Assist
You should inform the victim that help is on the
way for reassurance.

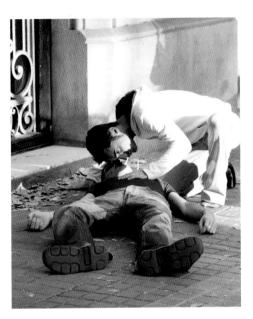

It is important to wrap the injured person in something
warm to try to maintain her body temperature.

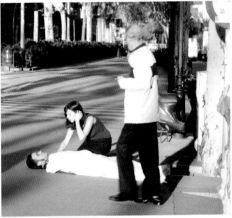

The pulse should be taken with two fingers against the
wrist. The thumb has its own pulse and should never
be used, since this could lead to confusion between the
pulse of the person taking it and that of the casualty.

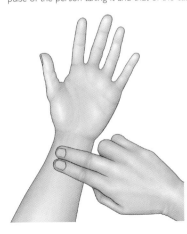

In a situation requiring first aid, the person assisting must be very conscious of two things:

- If they are sure what to do, they must take
  action, but it may be preferable to do nothing, because the help given may be unsuitable and aggravate the casualty's condition even further.

- Remaining clear-headed and acting calmly
  and quickly always inspires confidence in
  the casualty and helps you to perform the
  necessary techniques and procedures.

Basic rules of first aid

The aim of first aid treatment in an emergency is to improve the condition of the victim or, at the very least, to make sure the condition does not deteriorate. For this reason, it is important to know some basic rules so as to avoid errors and prevent the situation getting worse.

■ How do you know if the victim is breathing?

- Put your ear to the casualty's nose and try to detect his/her breathing.

- Try to detect breathing by placing the back of your hand over the casualty's nose.

- Place your hand gently against the chest to feel the heart beating.

- Place a mirror close to the nostrils and see if it becomes misty.

- The normal respiratory rate is 15 to 20 breaths per minute.

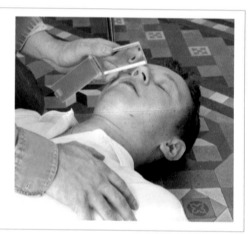

What should you do in an emergency?

- Follow the PAA rules: Protect, Alert, and Assist.
- If the casualty is conscious, ask them to accept your help, so as to reassure them.
- Maintain calm. This is always absolutely essential, as much for the person helping as for the sick or injured individual. If a sense of calm is communicated to the victim, this will considerably reduce their fear and convince them that there is little cause for alarm.

- If you are not completely sure of what to do, it is better to do nothing, since in this situation any action might exacerbate the problem.
- Make bystanders move back, so that, when medical assistance arrives, no obstruction is caused.
- Under no circumstances make any comment that might upset the casualty further.
- Examine the victim: take the pulse, see if she is breathing, in which case check the respiratory rhythm; confirm whether the airways (mouth and nose) are obstructed or not by blood, whether there is vomiting or discharge of other fluids, such as urine, etc.; examine the tongue.

Light-induced reflexes

When you shine a light into the person's eye, the pupil should contract.

If the opposite happens, this can be a sign of cardiac arrest.

If the pupil has already contracted, this can indicate a cerebral injury.

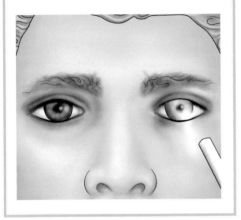

• See if the person is bleeding.

• If the victim has vomited and it is certain that there are not any skull, neck, or spinal fractures, move the head to one side to ease the functioning of their airways.

• Loosen the victim's clothing to avoid any constriction.

• Cover the victim with something warm (some clothing, a blanket, or similar, etc.), with the aim of maintaining the body temperature.

• If there are people nearby, try to find out from them how the accident happened.

• Ask if anyone around is a medical professional (a doctor, technical assistant, etc.) or a person with knowledge of first aid.

What not to do?

• Do not move the casualty, unless absolutely necessary (for example, when the victim is in a dangerous place).

• If you move the casualty, avoid any abrupt or unnecessary action.

• If there is any suspicion that the casualty has a fracture, do not move him, especially if there might be a spinal or cranial injury (in which case, the victim should be kept lying down and at rest).

• If the victim is unconscious, do not shake him, or try to give him liquids or medicines.

• Do not make any comments about the state of the casualty, even if you notice that the casualty is unconscious.

• Do not move from the site until medical help arrives.

• Never leave the casualty alone at any time.

• Do not administer any medicine.

• Do not provide alcohol, or coffee, or allow them to smoke.

• Do not touch wounds with your hands, your mouth or non-sterilized material (if necessary, use sterilized gauze, wherever possible).

• Do not blow on the wounds.

• Do not wash deep wounds (cover them only with sterile gauze).

• Avoid washing superficial wounds towards the inside, always do this with gentle movements towards the outside.

• Do not touch or move clotted blood.

• Do not try to sew up the wound.

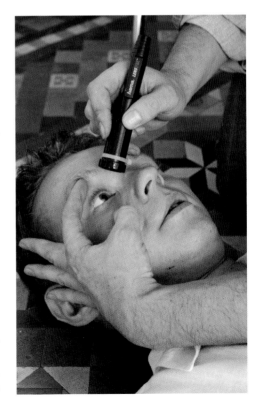

Limb reflexes

Pinch the inside flesh of an arm or leg. The absence of any response indicates that the person is deeply unconscious or has suffered a cardiac arrest. If they are only slightly unconscious, their limb will contract.

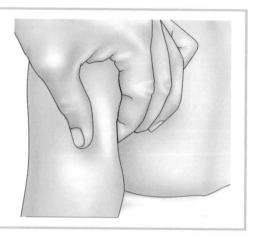

• Do not place cotton swabs over wounds or burns.

• Do not put band-aids directly over wounds.

• Do not remove gauze covering wounds abruptly.

• Do not apply wet bandages.

• Do not put alcohol on any part of the body.

Situations requiring urgent hospital treatment

In any of the following situations (which are extremely serious), the casualty should be taken swiftly to hospital if a means of transport is available:

• If you discover that the casualty has no pulse.

• When the casualty is not breathing or is having serious difficulty in doing so.

• If the bleeding is severe and extreme, or continues for more than 4 minutes.

• If you suspect that the casualty has appendicitis, or is in extreme danger (following a heart attack, brain hemorrhage, stomach perforation, drowning, or severe choking, etc.) and needs urgent treatment.

• If you detect poisoning.

• When the casualty is spatially and temporally disoriented and does not recognize family members, etc.

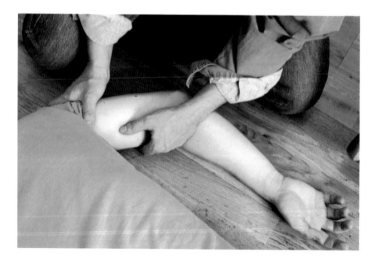

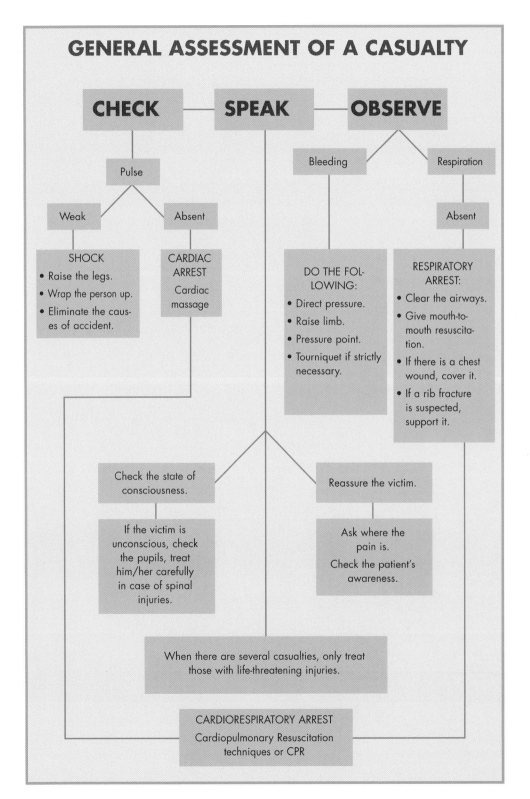

GENERAL ASSESSMENT OF A CASUALTY

CHECK — SPEAK — OBSERVE

Pulse

Weak

Absent

SHOCK
- Raise the legs.
- Wrap the person up.
- Eliminate the causes of accident.

CARDIAC ARREST

Cardiac massage

Bleeding

Respiration

Absent

DO THE FOLLOWING:
- Direct pressure.
- Raise limb.
- Pressure point.
- Tourniquet if strictly necessary.

RESPIRATORY ARREST:
- Clear the airways.
- Give mouth-to-mouth resuscitation.
- If there is a chest wound, cover it.
- If a rib fracture is suspected, support it.

Check the state of consciousness.

If the victim is unconscious, check the pupils, treat him/her carefully in case of spinal injuries.

Reassure the victim.

Ask where the pain is.
Check the patient's awareness.

When there are several casualties, only treat those with life-threatening injuries.

CARDIORESPIRATORY ARREST

Cardiopulmonary Resuscitation techniques or CPR

Emergency first aid kit

A first aid kit is necessary at home, at school, in the workplace, on vacation, when traveling, or camping. Its contents should therefore be kept in a small, portable box. Medicines are generally not included.

Essential material that a home kit should contain

- Oxygenated water
- Rubbing alcohol
- Mild antiseptic soap or solution
- Cotton swabs
- Sterile gauze
- Wet tissues for cleaning your hands.
- Analgesics (aspirin and acetaminophen (Tylenol))
- Antidiarrheic remedies
- Laxatives
- Antiseptic cream
- Cream for burns
- Antihistamine
- Tweezers
- Adhesive dressing tape
- Box of adhesive band-aids
- Sterilized gauze dressings (4x4 inches) (10x10 cm), in separate packages for cleaning wounds and dressing them afterwards
- Blunt-ended dressing scissors
- Thermometer
- Latex gloves

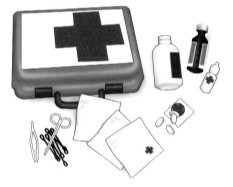

A first aid kit contains the necessary materials to give emergency assistance. Always bear in mind that the further away you are from a medical center, the more complete the first aid kit should be.

Home first aid kit

Since accidents at home may occur despite the many precautions taken, it is better to be prepared. The first aid kit should not be confused with the medicine chest or the place where drugs are kept. Medicines may require special storage conditions (a cool, dark and dry atmosphere, under lock and key), which may not be necessary for the first aid kit.

The kit should be kept in a well-marked location and never locked; at the same time, it

If you are on a course of treatment and envisage traveling abroad, it is advisable to bring medicines and health products in sufficient quantities for the whole trip, since it may be difficult and even impossible to obtain specific products in the country you are visiting.

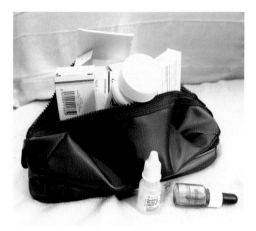

should be kept in a place outside the reach of children.

Some advice regarding the kit's location

• It should be in a visible place that is not locked, since its contents must be accessible.

• The container that makes up the kit should be plastic or metal.

• All the people who share the dwelling should be quite sure where the kit is kept.

• At intervals, you should check the expiration dates of the first aid material kept in it.

Some advice about drugs.

• Avoid storing a lot of drugs at home, since it becomes more difficult to keep control of them.

• Regular checks on the kit should be done every three or four months.

• Take out drugs that have expired or are no longer necessary.

• Discard drugs whose smell or color has changed—even if it is before their expiration date.

• Refrain from taking drugs whose original appearance has changed.

• Remember that expired drugs may no longer be effective; they may have toxic effects.

• Note down on each drug's box the date it was acquired and what uses are indicated for it.

Don't leave it too late to think about the health aspects of a journey. There are a number of things that should be planned in advance, such as visiting an international vaccination center. They will have detailed information about the necessary vaccines, the health conditions of the country being visited and the preventive measures that should be taken such as the use of repellents, antimalarial medication, etc.

• To avoid the possibility of self-harm, do not keep drugs that are left over from previous treatments prescribed by the doctor.

• Do not throw drugs in the trash bin. It is better to take them to the pharmacy or a recycling plant.

• Drugs and medical supplies should be kept in a place that is clean, dry, and cool, protected from sunlight and inaccessible to insects and animals. Some medicines should be kept in the refrigerator. Store them in their original packages.

• Medicine should not be kept in the bathroom or kitchen, since the frequent changes in humidity or temperature of these locations can destroy, degrade, or reduce the effectiveness of the medicines.

• Read the leaflet accompanying the drugs carefully. If the recommended storage temperature for

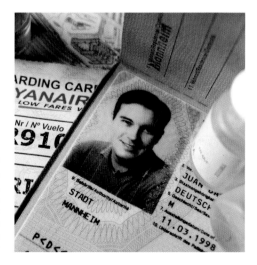

Travel kit contents

- Oxygenated water
- Rubbing alcohol
- Mild antiseptic soap or solution
- Cotton swabs
- Sterile gauze
- Wet tissues for cleaning your hands
- Analgesics
- Antidiarrheic remedies
- Laxatives
- Antiseptic cream
- Cream for burns

- Antihistamine
- Travel sickness medication
- Tweezers to extract splinters
- Adhesive dressing tape
- Box of adhesive band-aids
- Sterilized gauze dressings (4x4 inches) (10x10 cm), in separate packages for cleaning wounds and dressing them afterwards
- Blunt-ended dressing scissors
- Thermometer
- Latex gloves

Depending on the destination, you should also take with you:

- Tablets for disinfecting water
- Sunburn lotion
- Cream for insect stings
- Cream for local inflammations
- Activated carbon to absorb poisons ingested
- Sodium bicarbonate
- Small flask of ammonia

- Antimalarial medication
- Antibiotics
- Oral rehydration sachets
- International vaccination certificate
- Box of matches or lighter
- Flashlight
- Condoms

them is lower than the outside temperature, the storage conditions will be stated in the leaflet, with instructions such as "Store in the refrigerator in its own box" or "Do not refrigerate."

• Always keep medicines and first aid supplies in their original packages and with their corresponding instruction leaflets. In this way, you can always follow the instructions correctly and easily and have data available that allows you to identify the product in case it causes an undesirable reaction, such as allergy or poisoning.

• If you are traveling and need to take drugs with you, you must be careful about changes in temperature that might affect them; you should keep them in your hand baggage.

Travel kit

When traveling, especially in other countries, the drugs you normally take at home will likely not be available or go under a different name. Apart

from that, there is the problem that the doctor/druggist will not speak English and it may be difficult to find drugs for a minor complaint. For this reason, it is advisable before starting your journey, to prepare a specific kit suitable for your destination, the duration of the trip, and the type of activity.

The travel kit should be light and sturdy, and be kept in a very dry and cool place (avoiding areas under car windows or the upper parts of rucksacks). It is also advisable to take a few extra doses, in case of lost baggage, and prescriptions for the medicines being carried or a medical report to avoid possible problems at customs.

First aid kit for the car

It is just as important to have a first aid kit in the car as it is at home. Besides the contents of the basic first aid kit, you should include a flashlight and a blanket.

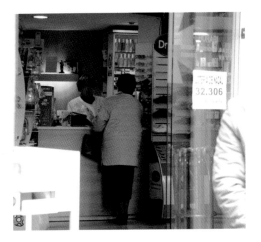

Your pharmacist is the most suitable and economical health expert to go to for advice about the contents of the kit and other questions prior to the journey.

The first aid kit at work

The contents of the first aid kit at work should be appropriate to the level of training of the person in charge of first aid. It is important that it is always kept in order, so that the people who use it find each item in its place.

▪ **Remember**

Some other general health advice regarding travel:

- If you wear eyeglasses, you should bring a replacement pair. It is advisable to bring prescription sunglasses.

- Those with specific health problems (having a pacemaker, suffering from diabetes, needing dialysis, etc.), are advised to take their medical details, as well as their health card and the medicines required for their treatment.

- If you are allergic to a medicine, carry a note giving clear information about this fact.

- If you are driving, heavy meals and alcohol should be avoided.

Don't forget that antihistamines, muscular relaxants, certain psychopharmaceutical drugs and some analgesics are contraindicated for driving.

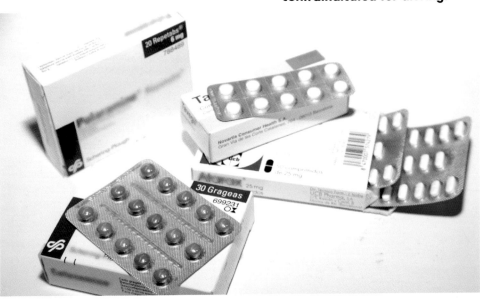

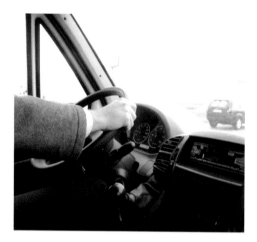

In first aid kits at work, the range of contents should be proportionate to the number of people who make up the organization and to the occupational risks. In some organizations, the accident frequency is high. For this reason, there should be a special area devoted to first aid and those in charge of giving assistance should generally be professionals. In these circumstances, there ought to be other drugs in the kit for treating sudden illnesses and they should be used exclusively by the specialized staff.

Contents of the car first aid kit

- In case no running water is available, the car kit should have saline or oxygenated water for washing wounds.
- Rubbing alcohol
- Mild antiseptic soap or solution
- Cotton swabs
- Sterile gauze
- Damp tissues for cleaning your hands
- Analgesics (aspirin and acetaminophen (Tylenol))
- Travel sickness pills
- Tweezers
- Adhesive dressing tape
- Box of adhesive band-aids
- Sterilized gauze dressings (4x4 inches) (10x10 cm) in separate packages for cleaning wounds and dressing them afterwards
- Blunt-ended dressing scissors
- Thermometer
- Latex gloves
- Flashlight
- Sections of material for splints and bandages
- Heat-insulating or thermal blanket
- List of emergency telephone numbers
- Disposable cups
- First aid manual

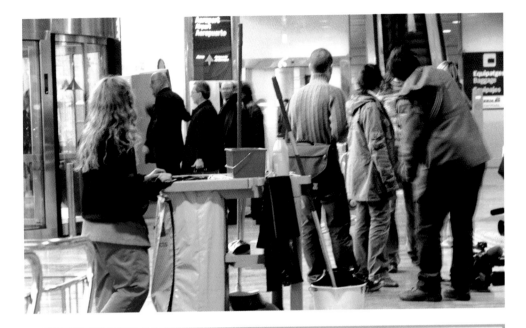

Contents of the first aid kit at work

- Oxygenated water
- Rubbing alcohol
- Iodine
- Mild antiseptic soap or solution
- Cotton swabs
- Sterile gauze
- Damp tissues for cleaning the hands
- Analgesics (aspirin and acetaminophen (Tylenol))
- Antidiarrheic remedies
- Laxatives
- Antiseptic cream
- Antihistamine
- Tweezers
- Adhesive dressing tape
- Box of adhesive band-aids
- Sterilized gauze dressings (4x4 inches) (10x10 cm) in separate packages for cleaning wounds and dressing them afterwards
- Blunt-ended dressing scissors
- Thermometer
- Latex gloves

- Eye patches
- Triangular provisional bandages.
- Thermal blanket
- Cardiopulmonary resuscitation mask (optional)
- Water or 0.9 percent saline solution in sealed disposable containers, in the absence of eye-wash fountains
- Cleaning tissues without alcohol, if soap and water is not available
- Plastic bags for used or contaminated first aid material
- Depending on the type of organization (in particular a factory or workshop using certain dangerous products, etc.), in addition to this essential equipment, it is advisable to include: a stretcher, oxygen, stitching equipment, cannula airway drainage tubing, syringes and hypodermic needles, splints for securing fractures, hemostatic pincers, an orthopedic collar, cold and warm compresses or a hot water bottle or icepack, a suction pump or bulb for extracting secretions, a tray for sterilizing instruments, a phonendoscope, a nasal gastric probe, and drugs strictly for medical use in emergencies

Fever

In the human body's struggle against certain illnesses, fever plays a fundamental role. So fever is an ally, not an illness.

Fever

Fever, also called hyperthermia or pyrexia, is defined as the abnormal increase in body temperature in response to attacks by organisms or by chemical or physical agents. The human body regulates the situation by means of fever, which normally is the first alarm signal indicating the presence of some problem.

• The normal average temperature in the human body is 98°F (36.7°C), although it can fluctuate between 97 and 99.32°F (36.1 and 37.4°C).

• The most important non-pathological factors that cause body temperature to vary are:

• An excessively hot or cold environment.
• Pregnancy during the first three months.
• Hormonal factors.
• Atmospheric changes taking place throughout the day.
• Changes in metabolism.
• Body temperature is normally lower in the morning and slightly higher in the evening.
• The temperature regulating system is controlled by the hypothalamus, somewhat like a thermostat.

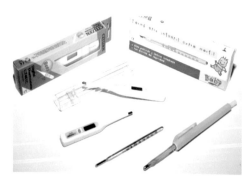

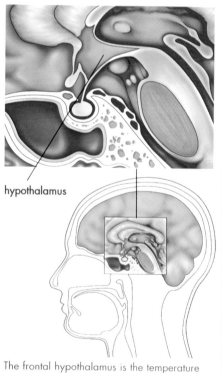

hypothalamus

The frontal hypothalamus is the temperature regulation center of the human body.

It causes your temperature to rise.

• If body temperature increases, it produces vasodilatation. (dilation of the blood vessels) and sweating, thus causing body temperature to fall. If body temperature falls, this causes vasoconstriction (narrowing of the blood vessels) to conserve the body's inner temperature.

Febrile syndrome

Fever is usually accompanied by a series of symptoms that can be grouped together under the term febrile syndrome.

- Cold sensation (shivering) in the initial phase and getting hot later
- Flushed face, shining eyes
- Discolored tongue
- Loss of appetite
- Tachycardia (acceleration of the pulse)
- Small quantity of urine, concentrated and dark in color
- Headache

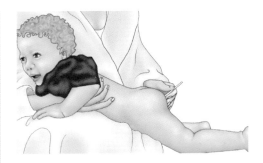

Main causes of fever

- The factors that may cause fever are highly diverse, since fever is a sign that something is not functioning correctly in the body.
  - Bacterial or viral infections.
  - Infections of the urinary tract.
  - Infections of the upper respiratory tract, such as tonsillitis, pharyngitis, or laryngitis.
  - Colds or flu.
  - Severe bronchitis.
  - Viral or bacterial gastroenteritis.
  - Throat inflammation and streptococcal pharyngitis.
  - Earache.
  - More rarely, it can be caused by illnesses such as pneumonia, appendicitis, tuberculosis and meningitis.

How do you take someone's temperature?

- Clean the thermometer with soap and water, or a little alcohol.
- Shake the thermometer firmly until the mercury that indicates the temperature has fallen to 96.8°F (36°C) or below. The most effective way of holding the thermometer is between the thumb and index finger.

Checking for fever by placing your hand over the patient's forehead is a very imprecise method that can give rise to frequent errors. To take someone's temperature, a clinical thermometer should always be used.

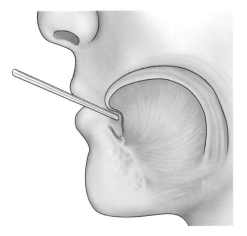
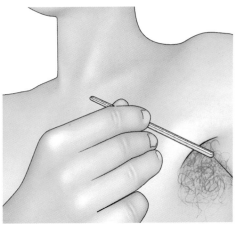

What should be done when someone has a fever?

If there are no evident problems and the fever is light:

- Drink a lot of liquids and rest.
- If you are uncomfortable or have muscular pain, it might be helpful to take an antipyretic, such as aspirin or acetaminophen (Tylenol).

In cases where the person with fever presents symptoms such as:

- Discomfort,
- Vomiting,
- Dehydration,
- Difficulty resting, the fever should be reduced.

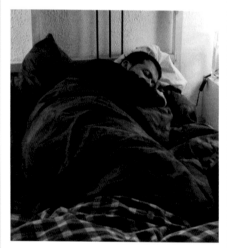

If the fever is light and not causing problems, it is recommended to drink a lot of liquids and to rest.

When the fever is high—101.3°F (38.5°C) or above— you should telephone the doctor. However, with children, it should be borne in mind that their temperature can easily reach high levels and then go down again in a few hours.

- To measure temperature orally:
  - Place the base of the thermometer under the tongue.
  - Tell the patient to close their mouth gently.
  - Wait 3 minutes.
  - read the temperature.
- To measure temperature in the armpit:
  - Place the base of the thermometer in the armpit.
  - Ask the patient to keep their arm in contact with their body.
  - Wait 4 minutes.
  - Add about 1 degree F (0.5 degrees C) to the value indicated by the thermometer.
- To measure temperature rectally:
  - Use a rectal thermometer (it has a larger base).
  - Apply Vaseline to the base.
  - Insert the base gently into the rectum.
  - Wait 3 minutes.
  - Subtract 1 degree F (0.5 degrees C) from the value indicated by the thermometer.
  - Do not forget to clean the thermometer with mild soap, water, and a little alcohol after each reading.

In the case of fever in a small child, call the doctor immediately:

- If they present symptoms, such as stiffness in the neck, confusion, irritability, or drowsiness.
- In a baby less than 6 months old, if they present symptoms of fever at any time.
- In an infant between 6 months and a year old, if they have a prolonged fever for more than 24 hours.
- If there is persistent fever above 102.9°F (39.4°C) one hour after commencement of treatment.
- If the fever lasts more than two days.
- Any child whose temperature remains above 102.9°F (39.4°C) should be examined by a doctor.

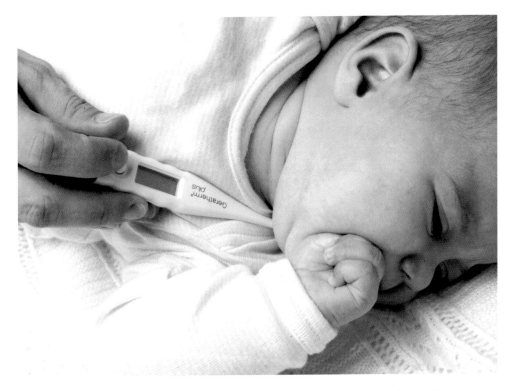

Fever-reducing medications should not be administered to babies less than 3 months old without first consulting a doctor.

If someone, especially someone of advanced age, mentions that they feel cold, you should take their temperature with a thermometer.

How to reduce fever

• Remove any excess bed coverings so as to create a comfortable and slightly cool environment.

• In the case of shivering, do not cover the person up anymore.

• If the room is excessively hot, use a fan.

• It is helpful to refresh the person using a sponge or cloths soaked in lukewarm water.

• Do not bathe them in cold water.

• Do not rub them with alcohol, since this causes more shivering, and may lead to another rise in temperature.

• Give them lots of liquids.

• Recommended medications for adults are:

– Ibuprofen.

– aspirin.

– acetaminophen (Tylenol)

What is hypothermia?

• When the body temperature descends dangerously low below 95°F (35°C), it is called hypothermia, which is a medical emergency in every case.

• What appears to be only a few degrees below normal temperature (98.6°F (37°C)) () can have serious effects on your health; for this reason, it is very important to detect symptoms in time.

What are the symptoms of hypothermia?

– Shivering.

– Sleepiness, confusion.

– Weak pulse and irregular heartbeat, which can lead to cardiac failure and death.

– Low blood pressure.

– Shallow breathing.

– Stiffness in the limbs.

The doctor must be called immediately if the fever continues without abating, and is accompanied by the following symptoms:

- Intense headache
- Stomachache
- Earache
- Pain when urinating
- Intense pain in the joints
- Stiffness in the neck
- Difficulty in breathing
- Inflamed throat

- Vomiting
- Diarrhea
- Dehydration
- The patient is in a confused state (they cannot answer simple questions such as: what is your name?, where do you live?, what month is it?)
- Convulsions

– Poor control of movement.
– Difficulty in communicating, poor reactions.

Preventing hypothermia.
What should you do if you need to spend a long time outdoors at low temperatures?
- Avoid consuming alcohol and smoking.
- Drink lots of liquids.
- Rest.
- If you think that the temperature is going to be extremely cold, or the wind strong, it is better to avoid going out at all. But if you have to:
- Avoid damp clothing.
- Do not wear clothing or footwear that is too tight and inhibits blood circulation.
- Wear several layers of clothing which is both waterproof and resistant to cold.
- Wear the following articles of clothing, in order to avoid loss of body temperature: mittens, two pairs of socks, one of cotton and the other wool, a scarf, and protection for the head and ears.

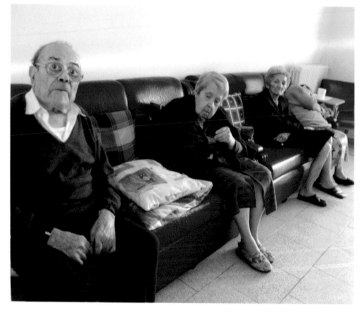

The people who are most likely to present symptoms of hypothermia are the elderly and children, people with nutritional problems, especially associated with the consumption of toxic substances, patients with chronic illnesses (cardiovascular, renal illnesses) or debilitating conditions (infections, tumors), people with thyroid or other metabolic problems (hypoglycemia), people who take certain drugs (barbiturates and sedatives), and people who work in the open air without adequate protection.

DEFINITION OF HYPOTHERMIA	TEMPERATURE	SIGNS AND SYMPTOMS
Light	>9.96°F (32.2°C)	Complaining of cold. Conscious." Normal arterial pressure. Shivering.
Moderate	80.06°F–89.96°F (26.7°C–32.2°C)	Intermittent shivering. Muscular stiffness. Midriasis (pupil dilation). Reduction in respiratory rate. Semiconscious.
Severe	< 80.06°F (26.70°C)	Limpness. Dyspnea. Ventricular fibrillation. Comatose state.

What should be done in cases of severe hypothermia?

• Alert the emergency medical services.

• If possible, remove the patient's clothing if it is damp and shelter them from cold, damp, rain, or wind.

• Alcohol should not be given. They should be given warm drinks (tea, hot milk, soups, etc.).

• Make sure the victim is taken speedily to hospital or to the nearest medical center, so that a suitable investigation and correct diagnosis can be made, and appropriate therapeutic measures can be commenced.

• If available, use a thermometer for hypothermia, given that normal thermometers do not register temperatures lower than 95°F (35°C) ().

• If the patient is unconscious, it is best to follow a series of specific rules for cardiovascular resuscitation:

– A good oxygen supply should be provided to the patient: mouth-to-mouth until the rescue teams arrive and later oxygen by the appropriate medical means: tube feed, etc.

– The use of cardiac massage may be required.

– If body temperature is below 86°F (30°C), the state of the patient is similar to that of death: muscular hypertonia, dilated and motionless pupils, no reflexes and undetectable blood pressure. In spite of this, you should persist with cardiac massage and mouth-to-mouth resuscitation. With the correct treatment, this state may be reversible without adverse consequences later.

• The most controversial aspect of hypothermia is identifying the best method for raising the body temperature of a patient who is suffering from moderate or severe hypothermia (temperature of about 89.6°F (32°C)). Recovery from hypothermia depends, to a great extent, on the previous health of the individual affected and on the factors that predisposed them to a reduction in their internal temperature. It is usually necessary to insert a tube into a vein and to administer warm liquids intravenously.

Intestinal complications: vomiting, diarrhea, constipation, and colic

The digestive system carries out the functions of ingestion, transport, digestion, absorption, and defecation. It is common for minor complications such as vomiting, diarrhea, constipation, and colic to occur. What should you do in the event of a stomach upset?

Vomiting

- Vomiting is an urgent need to expel the contents of the stomach.
- Sometimes, vomiting is a symptom of another illness, or may simply be a matter of a reflex action by the body towards food or drink that was unsuitable.

What should you do when a child is vomiting?
The most important thing is the way you treat the child. Vomiting can frighten young children (and parents, too) and exhaust children of any age. The key points are: keep the child calm and take the appropriate steps to prevent dehydration.

▪ What is an antiemetic drug?

- Antiemetic drugs are those that are used to prevent and alleviate nausea and vomiting. This type of drug limits the reflex action of vomiting caused by the central nervous system.

For children under the age of 1:
- Never give only water to a small child, unless the pediatrician specifically gives instructions to do so.

What should you do if vomiting occurs?

- Try to rest and lie down.
- It is very important to take liquids—in small quantities—to maintain the level of body hydration and thus avoid dehydration.
- In the case of babies, in whatever quantity is possible, the best thing is mother's milk. Babies who are bottle fed should take diluted formula.
- It's best not take a lot of liquid all at once, since it can have an adverse effect by straining the walls of the stomach and giving rise to further vomiting.
- If vomiting is very prolonged, a physician should be consulted, since this may be a signal of a more serious pathological condition.

• The child should be given small, but frequent quantities—2 or 3 teaspoons—of an oral electrolytic solution, sold in pharmacies, every 15 or 20 minutes approximately. Oral electrolytic solutions contain salts in the necessary concentration to restore what has been lost through vomiting or diarrhea, and also contain a little sugar. It is especially important for the liquids taken by small children to have a suitable amount of salt.

• Electrolytic solutions without any taste are best for small children.

• If the child is able to last more than a couple hours without vomiting, the dose of the solution should be increased gradually.

• If a child is only taking mother's milk and vomits (not just spits out, but vomits what appears to be their total intake) more than once, he or she should be breastfed from one breast only for 5 to 10 minutes every 2 hours. If the baby goes on vomiting, a doctor must be called. After 8 hours free from vomiting, you can go back to breastfeeding the baby from both breasts.

• When a baby less than 1 month old vomits everything that he or she ingests (not just spitting it out), the doctor should be called immediately.

For children of 1 year old or more:

• Children should be given clear liquids (it is better to avoid milk and other dairy products) in small quantities (1 or 2 spoonfuls) every 15 minutes. The clear liquids should include:
  – Water.
  – Oral electrolytic solutions.
  – Non-acidic fruit juices
  (for example, apple juice).

• Non-effervescent soft drinks at room temperature.

• If the child continues vomiting, begin with a smaller quantity of liquid (2 teaspoons) and continue with the instructions given earlier.

Vomiting in pregnant women

During pregnancy, women suffer from a series of physiological symptoms that cause discomfort, like constipation and acidity.

However, the most common complaint, which affects some 50–80 percent of pregnant women, is "morning sickness," which can begin to interfere with their daily activities if they are not given suitable treatment.

How can morning sickness be avoided?

Below are some recommendations for avoiding the sensation of nausea. If it does not get better, you should consult a physician. The nausea usually disappears around the third month of pregnancy.

Eat something dry and solid before getting up.

For example, some cookies or toast.

Do not eat fried food.

Do not eat spicy food.

Substitute your three main meals for five lighter snacks.

If you are losing weight as a result of vomiting,

or the vomiting is constant, consult a specialist.

More than half of pregnant women have unpleasant symptoms, but these disappear at the end of the first trimester.

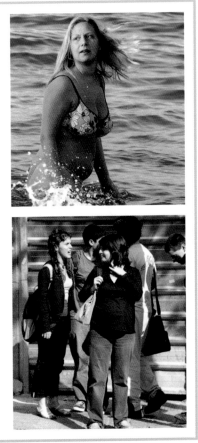

• If she hasn't vomited for 8 hours, she should gradually be introduced to light, soft foods. The child must not be forced to eat–she will say when she is hungry. Broth, clear soups (with noodles), mashed potatoes, rice, and bread are good choices.

• If the child doesn't vomit for 24 hours, she can gradually return to her normal diet. Wait for 2–3 days before giving her dairy products.

Vomiting and chemotherapy

Those who are about to start chemotherapy are apt to be very worried about its side effects, of which the most common is nausea and vomiting. Each individual reacts differently to the medication administered during chemotherapy, and also to each type of chemotherapy. Vomiting usually occurs several days after the patient has undergone the first treatment sessions.

General suggestions for avoiding nausea

In order to prevent or reduce the sensation of nausea and vomiting while receiving chemotherapy, here are some suggestions:

• On the day you are going to receive chemotherapy, do not eat big meals.

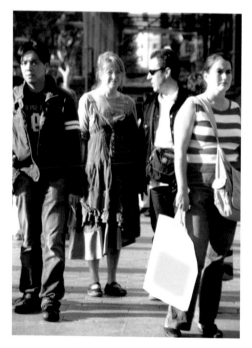

■ Why does chemotherapy produce side effects?

• Chemotherapy is a pharmacological oncological treatment that is used for a large number of cancers. This type of medication interrupts cell reproduction (it is cytotoxic) or inhibits their development (cytostatic) and its side effects derive from the way it acts upon healthy cells. In addition to that, it affects the central nervous system, causing nausea and vomiting.

• Do not consume alcohol.

• Do not eat your favorite foods on the day you receive chemotherapy, since, if you feel bad afterwards, you may easily come to hate this type of food.

• Consult the doctor about the kinds of food that help to prevent nausea and vomiting. There are many kinds, so that if one does not suit you, you can try another.

If nausea occurs, you should loosen your clothing to make you feel better; your room should be aired, bright light and loud noise should be avoided, and you should try to breathe deeply. If in the end you vomit, it is best to maintain a positive attitude; vomiting is simply a side effect of the medication and in no way means that the cancer is winning the battle.

Diarrhea

• Diarrhea is characterized by the sudden evacuation of watery, runny feces.

• Diarrhea in adults is usually moderate and gets better quickly.

• In babies, however, diarrhea can be a symptom of other more serious pathological conditions, and they also run the risk of becoming dehydrated more quickly than adults.

• The most frequent cause of diarrhea is a light viral infection.

There are many types of chemotherapy and new treatments are being developed that do not cause nausea and vomiting as a side effect.

What should be done if diarrhea occurs?

• Given that diarrhea is generally moderate and does not cause further complications, if you follow various recommended steps at home, it is possible to reduce the continual bowel evacuations.

• If the symptoms last for more than three days, a physician should be consulted.

• The general advice to be followed at home is:

– Maintain the level of body hydration. Take soups, juices, water, tea or soft drinks.

– After one day, start to include solid foods gradually, like boiled rice or toast.

– Avoid the consumption of dairy products, alcohol, caffeine, or spicy food.

– Do not take anti-diarrhea medication, unless prescribed by a doctor.

Diarrhea in travelers

• Sometimes, people who have visited an exotic country suffer a severe bout of diarrhea during the journey or on their return.

• The main cause is infection.

• The treatment is similar to that of common diarrhea, although, if the symptoms persist for

▪ You must call the doctor if:

• the feces contain blood or pus.

• the diarrhea has lasted more than 48 hours.

• you are suffering intense abdominal pain .

• the diarrhea is accompanied by vomiting that prevents maintenance of the optimal level of hydration.

• you have traveled recently to an exotic country.

Diarrhea affects between 20 and 50 percent of people who travel to tropical and subtropical zones in Africa, Latin America, and Southeast Asia.

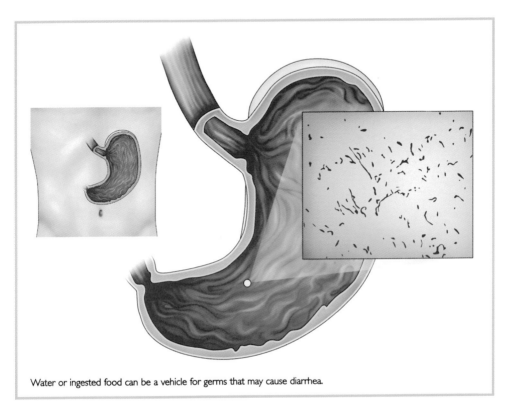

Water or ingested food can be a vehicle for germs that may cause diarrhea.

◾ How do you know if a baby is dehydrated?

It's easy to tell if a baby's diarrhea is causing dehydration. Here are some symptoms:
• Does he have dry eyes?
• Is he crying less than usual?
• Is his mouth dry?
• Are his diapers less moist than usual?
• Is he irritable?
If the answer is yes, the baby may have symptoms of mild dehydration, and you should maintain his hydration level by administering sufficient quantity of liquids.

more than three days, you should visit the doctor immediately and inform him or her that you have recently visited an exotic country.

How can you prevent diarrhea when traveling?
During the trip, you should take extra precautions with food and drink:
– Avoid food containing raw eggs.
– Do not drink running water, only bottled water.
– Do not use ice cubes in drinks, unless they have been made with bottled water.
– Do not get food from street stalls, since it probably does not meet the required standards of food safety.

Diarrhea in babies
• Diarrhea in babies must be controlled very carefully, given that they are very prone to suffer from dehydration, which could significantly worsen their state of health.
• Diarrhea in babies is generally caused by a virus and they recover quickly. Even so, you

should follow a series of recommended steps for avoiding discomfort in the child.

What should you do when a baby has diarrhea?
• Do not worry if they lose their appetite, although you must try to encourage them to take liquids. Continue with breast or bottle-feeding, with the aim of making them take liquid frequently in small quantities.
• In order to restore the sodium and potassium that they may have lost through diarrhea, hydration solutions for the child can be obtained from the pharmacy.
• Maintain a high level of hygiene: clean all their toys and wash your hands before coming into contact with the child.
• If the baby is on solid foods, give him light meals, like white rice and soups. Avoid fatty foods.

How do you know if a baby is dehydrated?
It's very easy to tell if a baby's diarrhea is causing dehydration. Here are some symptoms:
• Does he have dry eyes?
• Is he crying less than usual?
• Is his mouth dry?
• Are his diapers less moist than usual?
• Is he irritable?
If the answer is yes, the baby may have symptoms of mild dehydration, and you should maintain his hydration level by administering sufficient quantity of liquids.

Constipation
Constipation occurs when evacuation of feces is infrequent, or defecation becomes difficult.
• Each person has his own rhythm of intestinal evacuation, but on average, you can say that con-

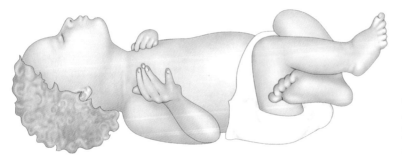

When a baby suffers diarrhea, you should change his diapers frequently to avoid skin irritation.

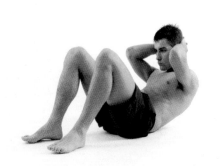

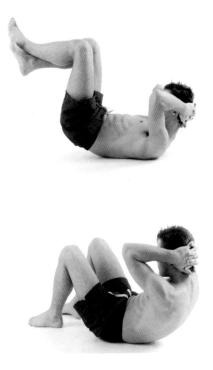

stipation is present when the frequency of evacuation is less than three times a week.

• Normally, it occurs along with changes in eating habits, or when traveling.

What should you do if you are constipated?

• You should follow three principal rules to improve bowel movement. In the first place, change your diet, then increase physical exercise, and finally, establish a regular evacuation rhythm.

• If this advice is followed and the constipation does not improve, you should consult a physician so that he can prescribe some laxative medication.

In order to ease bowel movement, it is very important to include fiber in your diet.

Do physical exercise

Abdominal exercises are very helpful if you suffer from constipation.

How to do these exercises:

• Go to a comfortable place, lie on your back, make sure that your back is in full contact with the ground and place your hands behind your neck.

Diet for constipation

• If fiber is included in your diet, it helps the intestine with digestion, thus helping to prevent constipation.

• To increase the beneficial effect of the fiber, it should be consumed with a lot of water.

• The main sources of fiber in foods for the human body are:

• Green vegetables.

• Fresh fruit.

• Bran.

• Whole grain cereals.

• Other dietary habits to prevent constipation are:

• Drink more than two liters of water a day.

• Take prune juice when going to bed.

• Avoid foods with little fiber, like sugar.

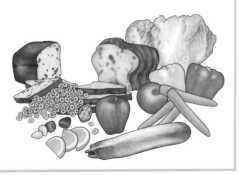

Constipation

TABLE OF RECOMMENDED FOODS AND THOSE NOT RECOMMENDED	
RECOMMENDED	**NOT RECOMMENDED**
Dairy products Milk, yogurt, and other dairy products with low fat content.	**Dairy products** Condensed milk, milk chocolate, or cream yogurt.
Meat All types of meat in moderation.	**Meat** Processed meat, offal, meat with a high fat content.
Fish All types of fish in moderation.	**Fish** Pickled, canned, or smoked fish.
Eggs As with meat and fish, in moderation.	**Cereals** White bread, chocolate cookies; cereals with cream, or a lot of sugar.
Cereals Preferably whole grain (bread, muesli).	**Rice** Avoid it but if eaten, it should be combined with green vegetables.
Green vegetables and garden produce They are all permitted, unless they cause flatulence. Eat one portion of salad daily.	**Vegetables** Not to be cooked with processed meats or pork fat.
Fruit Any fruit apart from those types in the non-recommended group.	**Green vegetables** Avoid green vegetables that produce gas, such as: leeks, cabbage, cauliflower, broccoli, peppers and cucumber, and also onions and radishes.
Drink Consume more than two liters of water a day, herbal infusions, fruit juices (preferably with pulp).	**Fruit** Lemon, apple, grapefruit, quince, peaches in syrup, pineapple in syrup and other canned fruit.
Fat Olive oil and sunflower oil are best consumed with salads, but not with fried products (this same advice applies to butter and margarine).	**Drink** Lemon juice, grapefruit juice, alcoholic drinks.

Some advice to stop a baby crying:

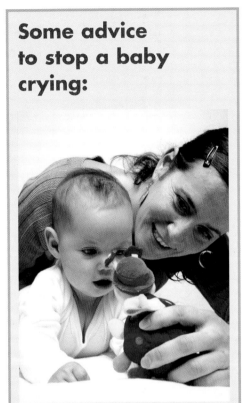

- Feeding a baby sitting down or burping him requently can help to avoid colic caused by swallowing air when feeding.

- Calm the child down holding him in your arms, rocking him, giving him gentle pats or giving him a gentle stomach massage.

- A baby who is desperate to nurse or complains immediately after having the bottle, probably needs to feed more.

- The pacifier may also help to settle him down.

- If the child is very agitated, perhaps a bath in lukewarm water will calm him down or maybe change his clothing and diaper.

• Raise your shoulders and upper body in the direction of your knees very gently. During this movement, breathe in softly.

• Point your head toward your knees rather than upward.

• Maintain this position for a second, then return slowly and gently to your starting position, breath-ing out at the same time. Repeat the exercise about 20 times a day. To be effective, abdominal exercises have to be done regularly and consistently. In this way you do not have to overexert yourself. The regular exercise is a way of training your body.

Establishing bowel rhythm

• When the reflex desire to relieve yourself occurs, do not stifle it; go to the toilet immediately.

• Also it is helpful to accustom the body to evacuate everyday at a set time.

• Set aside the necessary time for going to the toilet; stress and being in a hurry make it harder to develop the defecation reflex.

What is a kidney stone?

Kidney stones are composed of substances that are normally found in urine, but in a concentrated and solidified form. They can be of different sizes, from very small to more than an inch in diameter.

Indigestion

Digestion is a very slow process that becomes prolonged when too much food or food that is excessively rich in fat or fiber is ingested. In producing more acids to help digestion, the intestinal tract swells. Another form of indigestion is that which produces swelling of the abdomen. This occurs when the stomach feels too full and usually causes flatulence.

To reduce these unpleasant symptoms:

• Have papaya or fresh pineapple as a dessert, since they contain papain and bromelain respectively, enzymes that help in the digestion of proteins.

• Do not have an excess of meat, particularly ham and processed meats, and other foods that are rich in fat. It is better to eat turkey and game birds in season, which are easier to digest than lamb or duck (containing much more fat).

• Replace coffee with digestive infusions (chamomile, mint, fennel, cumin, or sage).

• If you know in advance that you are going to have a "special meal," this should be compensated for by ensuring that the rest of the day's meals are lighter than usual.

Nausea and vomiting

Whether as a result of consuming food in a poor state of preservation or of excessive alcohol, vom-

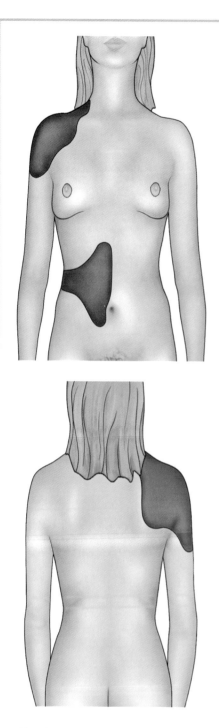

The pain caused by bilious colic is located in the right side of the abdomen, although it can extend as far as the shoulder.

iting is a way for the body to get rid of a toxic element. After vomiting and to avoid dehydration, it is essential to take in a sufficient amount of liquid, but it is better to wait 1–2 hours before having anything to drink.

As long as the vomiting has stopped, you can begin to have solid food. Dry foods are easier on the stomach: toast, matzos, etc. Certain homemade remedies help: for example a ginger infusion (slice and crush it, add one soup-spoonful for each cup of water and then boil it for 3–5 minutes) is ideal for combating indigestion with accompanying nausea, vomiting, travel sickness, and for eliminating gases.

▗▘ What should be done in the event of nephritic colic?

- Rest in bed.
- Apply heat to the painful area.
- Take a hot bath, at 97–98.5°F (36–37°C)).
- Take an analgesic to alleviate the pain.
- If the pain lasts more than three hours, call a doctor.

Colic

Colic in babies
- Colic is a common problem with nursing babies, who, in spite of being healthy, have periods of inconsolable crying, apparently caused by abdominal pain.
- Generally, colic occurs a few weeks after birth and disappears when the baby reaches four months.
- If the baby does not settle down, does not gain weight and has fever, he should be taken to a doctor immediately.

How can colic in babies be avoided?
- Feed the baby more frequently and in smaller quantities.
- If the baby takes powdered milk, try another brand, perhaps soy formula.
- Try to keep the baby's bottle at body temperature.
- If the baby feeds from the bottle very rapidly,

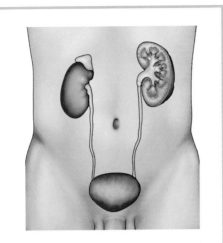

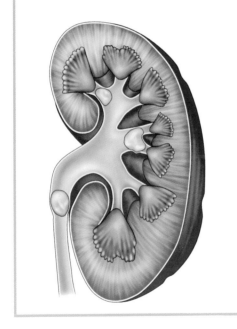

Renal colic is very common, affecting more than 10 percent of the middle-aged population. It is more frequent in men with sedentary jobs or life styles.

use a bottle with a smaller hole in the teat to try to make him feed more slowly.

Bilious colic

• This is caused by spasmodic contractions of the bilious ducts or gallbladder.

• Women are more prone to suffer this type of pain, especially after the age of 40, although it can also occur in men, and at any age.

What should be done in the event of colic?

• Some suggestions for alleviating the pain caused by colic:

– Make the patient lie down immediately.

– Make them take an analgesic to relieve the pain.

– Place hot compresses on the painful area.

– If the pain lasts for more than three hours, call a physician.

– As a preventive measure, cholesterol levels should be controlled.

Nephritic colic

• When a kidney stone is on its way out, it causes a blockage of the urine in the kidney, which produces a very severe and sharp pain in the area of the kidneys, possibly extending to the abdomen. It does not usually cause fever.

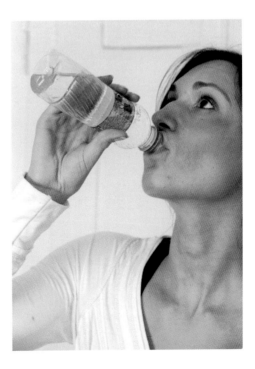

As a preventive measure and as a general rule, it is helpful to drink a lot of water every day, increasing the quantity during hot weather. At the same time, people with a tendency to suffer frequent bouts of renal colic should have metabolic-mineral tests to ascertain the cause of the colic.

How bile stones are formed and removed

• When a chemical imbalance occurs in the composition of bile, stones form, which may get caught in the bile ducts, or in the bladder itself. The bile stone is extracted using the technique of endoscopy. First, the stone is located using X-rays, and it is then removed with a laser.

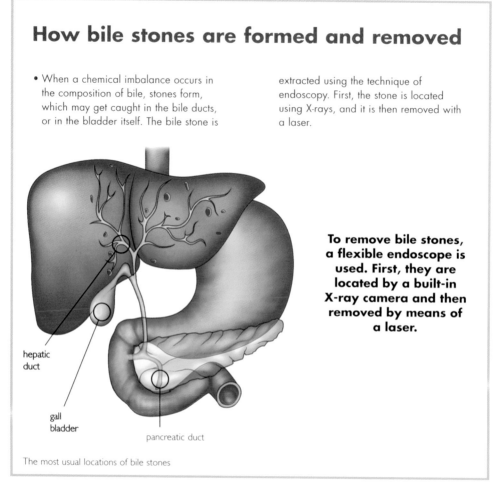

To remove bile stones, a flexible endoscope is used. First, they are located by a built-in X-ray camera and then removed by means of a laser.

hepatic duct

gall bladder

pancreatic duct

The most usual locations of bile stones

Flatulence

This is caused by an excess of gases in the intestine, producing intestinal spasms and abdominal distension (swelling of the abdomen). It can be a result of abrupt changes in diet, eating too fast and swallowing too much air while chewing, an excessive consumption of carbohydrates (rice, pasta, potato, bread, cereals, cookies, etc.), the use of antibiotics that disturb the balance of the intestinal micro-organisms, or the ingestion of foods that produce flatulence (foods creating gas and producing odors). In order to prevent these uncomfortable symptoms, you should do the following:

• Chew food well, eat and drink slowly.

• Use aromatic herbs that help digestion (rosemary, sage, thyme, fennel, hyssop, caraway, summer savory).

• Avoid very fatty foods and strong sauces.

• Substitute normal coffee for decaffeinated and replace tea with infusions of mint, sage, or fennel, or add a few grains of green aniseed, fennel, or cumin to a chamomile infusion, since they help digestion. Mint relaxes the muscles of the colon (large intestine), helping to alleviate the unpleasant build-up of gases.

• Yogurt contains bacteria that help to keep the intestinal micro-organisms in balance, and is thus especially recommended.

To aid digestion

• Eat slowly and in a relaxed way, spending at least 20–30 minutes for each meal.

• Chew your food well; do not forget that the digestion of many foods (cereals, potatoes, and vegetables) begins in the mouth.

• Do not use condiments (strong spices, mustard, etc.), which irritate the gastric mucus lining and increase stomach acidity. Food can be seasoned with digestive aromatic herbs (grains of aniseed, caraway, fennel, thyme, sage, cumin, cardamom, etc.). You can also have digestive or relaxing infusions of chamomile, lemon balm, white hawthorn, lime blossom, licorice, and fennel, etc.

• It is better not to drink a lot during meals or just afterwards, since this dilutes the gastric juices and delays digestion.

• Avoid large portions, very hot or very cold food and drinks, fried food, tobacco, abuse of alcohol and drinks that are stimulants (coffee and tea) and an excess of sugar. Do not take drugs that irritate the stomach.

• If you cannot resist the temptation to eat a particular dish or dessert, you must be reasonable and compensate in other ways: so if the starter is fatty or rich in calories, you should choose grilled or baked fish for the next course accompanied by salad or vegetables, and, fresh fruit for dessert.

• Do not lie down immediately after meals. The emptier your stomach is before a nap, the better.

It is advisable to drink 2 to 3 liters of water a day and maintain a healthy balanced diet .

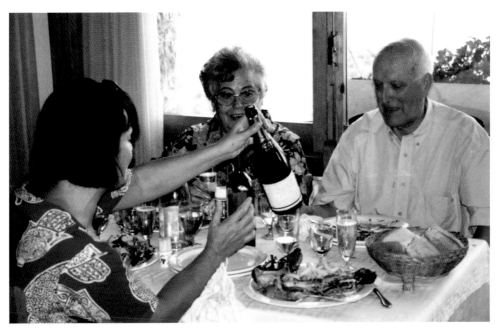

Headaches and migraine

Headaches are a common complaint: ninety percent of the population have suffered from them at least once. Headaches often cause anxiety to the sufferer, since they can have a non-pathological origin, such as stress or fatigue, or are the symptom of a more serious condition.

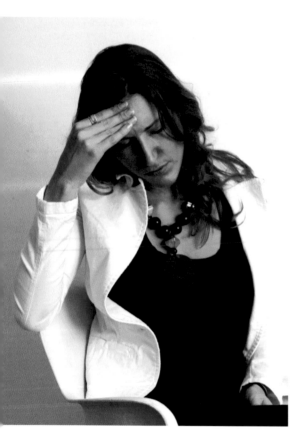

Types of headache

At present, more than 150 types of headache have been identified, although the most common are tension headaches and migraines. Given that the treatment for each type of headache is different, it is very important to distinguish between the different kinds.

Tension headache

This type of headache is very common in people with a heavy workload or a lot of family worries, and it causes considerable stress. It also occurs in people with an obsessive nature or those who are perfectionists. This type of headache may conceal a more serious condition, such as depression or other psychological problems.

The most common characteristics of a tension headache are:

• Oppressive pain (a feeling of pressure in the head).

Most migraines are characterized by pain in one or both sides of the head, nausea, dizziness, and photophobia.

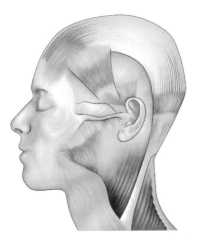

A tension headache is generally caused by tension in the muscles of the face, the neck and shoulders .

• They are of moderate intensity. Someone who suffers from this type of headache can continue with their work or their daily tasks.

• There is no associated nausea or vomiting.

• These headaches do not cause photophobia or phonophobia.

What is photophobia?

Photophobia is a very common symptom in headaches of a migraine type. It consists of an over-sensitivity of the eyes to light. For this reason, individuals who have migraine like to remain in the dark.

What is phonophobia?

In contrast to photophobia, phonophobia is an over-sensitivity to sound. Individuals who suffer from phonophobia as one of their headache symptoms are troubled by the slightest sound.

Migraines.

Migraines are normally localized in one side of the head and their intensity varies between moderate and intense. People who suffer from migraine find that their daily activities are interrupted when they experience an attack. Women are more prone to this type of headache.

The most important characteristics of migraines are:

• Pain localized in one side of the head, and more rarely in both sides.

• Pulsating pain (the pain is not continuous).

• Presence of photophobia and phonophobia.

• Presence of nausea and vomiting.

• Increases with exercise, coughing, or when turning the head to one side.

• One in five people experience aura.

What is aura?

One in five people who suffer migraine, are able to predict their next attack by experiencing aura. The main characteristics of aura are:

• Seeing sparkling lights.

• Faint blindness in one eye.

• Tunnel vision.

• More rarely, numbness in part of the body.

The aura appears approximately one hour before migraine pain and lasts normally up to 3 or 4 minutes, never more than one hour.

How to prevent migraines

For people who suffer from migraine, it is very important to follow an orderly sleep pattern and a healthier life style, together with other general recommendations:

• Do not smoke.

• Do not drink alcohol.

• Establish a daily sleep routine: sleep the same amount each day and go to bed at the same time each day.

• Learn to practice relaxation exercises that help to release muscular tension.

• Eat a healthy diet and avoid skipping meals.

• Do not eat foods that cause headaches; be wary of wine, beer, cheese, chocolate, nuts, processed foods, and meats.

■ What should be done in the event of a tension headache?

• First, you should reduce or eliminate the causes of it.

This can be done in different ways:

• Learn to cope with stress.

It is very helpful to learn meditation and mental relaxation techniques.

• Try to maintain a good posture while working.

• Get enough sleep and rest.

• If these measures do not work, take an analgesic, such as aspirin or ibuprofen.

What should you do in the event of a migraine attack?

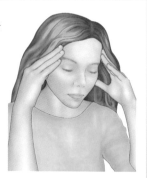

- It is very important to deal with the symptoms as soon as possible. People who suffer from frequent migraine are generally able to detect the early symptoms, being familiar with the developmental stages of such a pathological attack, and are thus able to avoid extreme pain.
- When migraine pain has already begun, you can do the following:
- Relax in a place that is free from intense light and noise.
- If the attack is accompanied by nausea and vomiting, drink a lot of liquid.
- Place a cold cloth over your head.
- If the pain becomes more intense or if you suffer more than three attacks a month, you might consult a doctor. He can prescribe drugs that act upon the blood vessels in the brain and relieve the pain.

- Avoid mediciness that cause headaches (consult the pharmacist), such as oral contraceptives and hormones.

Natural remedies against headaches
Although conventional remedies, like aspirin and ibuprofen, are effective in most cases, many people want to try natural remedies, due to the side effects occasionally caused by the usual drugs—in particular, of a gastric or intestinal nature. There are several alternative therapies.

Here are some of them:
- In the event of a tension headache, given that the underlying factor is stress, you can try to alleviate it through massage, yoga, relaxation techniques, or acupuncture.
- Magnesium is very helpful in reducing and helping to eliminate stress. It acts by relaxing the blood vessels, reducing the risk of pain. Patients who have migraine suffer from constriction of the blood vessels.
- In various clinical studies, it has been demonstrated that the consumption of vitamins B2 and B6 helps to reduce the pain caused by tension headaches and migraines.
- The herb kava (found in any herbal store) has a dual effect: it relieves anxiety and stress, and relaxes muscles. It is therefore highly effective for tension headaches.
- Ginger alleviates the nausea that occurs during migraine attacks.
- Lavender is traditionally used to alleviate tension headaches.

Where can I obtain vitamin B2?

- Vitamin B2, also known as riboflavin, is found in lean meat, eggs, vegetables, nuts, and milk, and their derivatives.

Where can I obtain vitamin B6?

- Vitamin B6 is found in beans, dried fruit, vegetables, eggs, meat, fish and whole grains (bread and cereals).

Earache

Earache, sometimes called otalgia, is one of the most troublesome common ailments. The pain is caused by the inflammation of the middle and outer structures of the ear. An infection, called otitis, is the most common cause of this pain. Otitis media results from infection of the middle ear, while otitis externa results from infection in the outer ear.

Anatomy of the ear

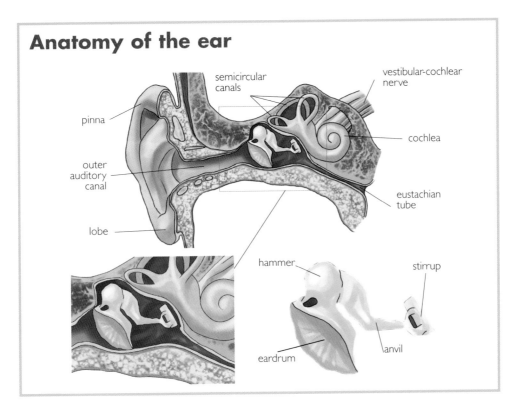

semicircular canals

vestibular-cochlear nerve

pinna

cochlea

outer auditory canal

eustachian tube

lobe

hammer

stirrup

eardrum

anvil

Earache

Otitis media is the inflammation and/or infection of the middle ear. It can be of two types: severe or chronic. Severe otitis media is usually caused by viral or bacterial infections, whereas the chronic variety results from a blockage in the eustachian tube, due to infections, allergies, or blows to the ear.

The outer ear is formed by the external auricular chamber and the outer ear canal, and closed off by the eardrum. The middle ear consists of the chain of little bones and the eustachian tube, which are a contact link between the middle ear and the pharynx.

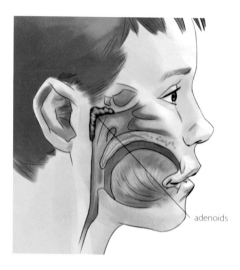

adenoids

How can chronic otitis media be alleviated?

- As with severe otitis media, the objective is to minimize the symptoms and reduce the infection.

- Normally, antibiotics are prescribed (if the infection is bacterial and not viral). This is a long-term type of treatment, given orally or in the form of drops to be applied in the ear.

- Other methods consist of extracting the adenoids by means of surgery, with the aim of removing the obstruction in the eustachian tube.

- The eardrum can also be opened surgically to drain off possible liquids that have accumulated.

Chronic otitis media

This inflammation or infection of the ear occurs when the eustachian tube is blocked or remains blocked for long periods.

- The eustachian tube extends between the middle ear and the pharynx. It can become blocked because of allergies, infections, blows, or inflammation. The blockage can also be caused by an ear infection that has not cleared up, or by repeated infections, such as mastoiditis.

Severe external earache

Otitis externa, also called "swimmer's ear," is caused by a skin infection that covers the outer

What is the mastoid apophysis?

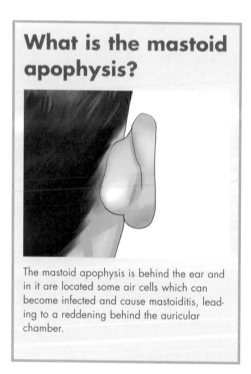

The mastoid apophysis is behind the ear and in it are located some air cells which can become infected and cause mastoiditis, leading to a reddening behind the auricular chamber.

How can severe otitis media be alleviated?

The main objective is to reduce the pain, cure the infection, and prevent complications. This type of infection generally recovers by itself without the need for drugs. You are advised to:

- Apply analgesic drops in the ear, sold in drugstores without the need for prescription.

- Take analgesics, such as acetaminophen (Tylenol) and ibuprofen, to relieve the pain.

- If a child with severe otitis media is under two years old, or has fever, or if his condition does not improve after 24 hours, it will be necessary to use antibiotics, although only when strictly necessary. Consult your doctor about which type of antibiotic is most suitable.

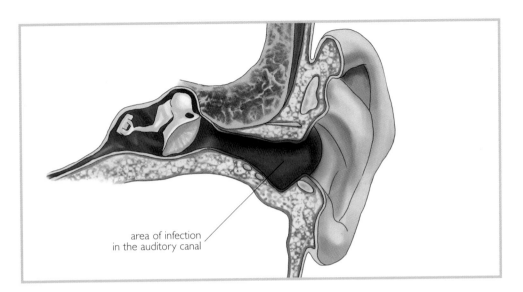

area of infection
in the auditory canal

auditory canal. It usually occurs in children, when their ears have been wet for long periods. The children feel stinging and pain in the auditory canal. It is often accompanied by a clear secretion.

How to cure swimmer's ear

It is helpful to clean the whole auditory chamber well and not allow it to be in contact with water. Consult a physician or druggist regarding antibiotics to combat the infection, and corticosteroids to reduce the stinging and inflammation. It is advisable to apply the drops generously so they can

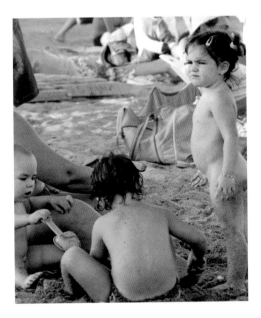

Earache when traveling by air: aerotitis

- More than a third of those who fly have unpleasant auditory symptoms, according to statistics. The most usual advice to follow to avoid earache during a flight is to chew gum for the whole flight, not just at take-off and landing. If someone suffers from auditory congestion, they should avoid flying.

penetrate the whole auditory duct more effectively. If the pain is very intense, analgesics like acetaminophen (Tylenol) or aspirin can be taken, or heat can be applied to the painful area.

Other causes of earache

Sometimes, earache is a sign of another illness or underlying complication. This can happen in the following situations:

- With certain dental problems, such as the emergence of wisdom teeth.
- Problems in the joints, such as torticollis.
- Complications in the lymphatic structures (ganglia).

Food poisoning

Food poisoning occurs when we ingest food contaminated by bacteria or containing substances that are toxic for the body. The main types of bacteria that cause food poisoning are Escherichia coli, Staphylococcus aureus, and Salmonella typhi.

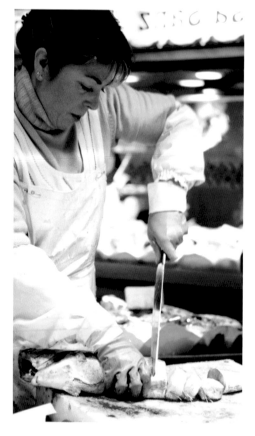

Correct handling of food, following basic rules of hygiene, prevents poisoning and infections from food.

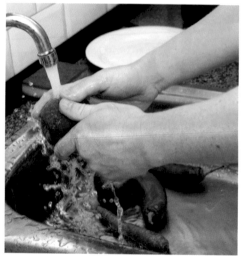

It is very important to wash fruits and vegetables before consuming them in order to remove the remains of pesticides.

Types of food poisoning

Food can be contaminated in three ways:

• **Biological contamination.** This occurs when food is contaminated by living agents (bacteria, viruses, and parasites). The altered state of the food is not clearly visible (no change in odor or in color), so that it does not arouse suspicion.

• **Chemical contamination.** This occurs when food is contaminated by chemical substances, for example, fish, through marine con-

How does food become contaminated by germs?

Generally, food is contaminated by germs when correct rules for handling it are not followed:

- If people cough or sneeze over it.
- If it is handled with dirty hands or fingernails.
- If people touch it after going to the toilet.
- If it is washed in unclean water.
- If it is not in a container and insects are allowed to settle on it.
- If it is handled with dirty equipment (cloths, cutlery, etc.).

tamination, and in fruits and vegetables through the use of pesticides.

- **Physical contamination.** This is usually due to the presence of substances extraneous to the food: pieces of bone, feathers, stones, plastic, staples, wood, glass, etc.

What factors favor the spread of germs?

- Temperature. Germs can develop at a range of temperature from between 50 and 140°F (10 and 60°C), although their ideal temperature for reproduction is around 98.6°F (37°C), which corresponds to the temperature of the human body.
- Level of humidity. You are less likely to find germs in products that contain little water, since germs grow more easily in the presence of water or humidity.
- Nutrition content. If a food is rich in proteins and other nutrients, this favors the growth of micro-organisms.
- Time. Food should be stored cold, or prepared and served immediately. If not, the time that the food has been left unchilled will help germs to spread, for example if it has spent a long time between being prepared and served.

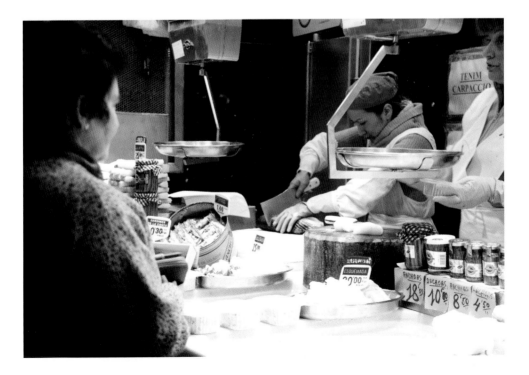

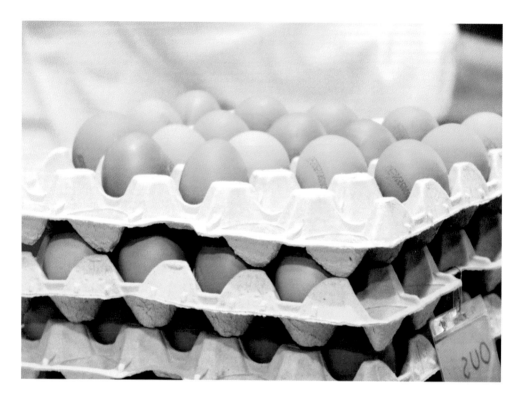

What are the main symptoms of food poisoning?

Fever. Fever is an alarm signal given by the body to warn that a pathogen is attacking body tissue; in this case, the digestive system. If food poisoning is suspected, body temperature should be measured with a thermometer.

• **Diarrhea.** In the case of food poisoning, this is severe. If the poisoning is at an advanced stage, the diarrhea may be accompanied by blood.

• **Vomiting.** This is another of the body's alarm signals.

• **Other symptoms.** There are toxins that act upon the central nervous system and cause headaches, sickness, instability, etc.

> If the person has fever symptoms only, it is impossible to know whether you are dealing with an infection or poisoning.

What should be done in a case of food poisoning?

• **Fever.** If the fever is light, it is better to let it follow its natural course, since the increase in body temperature will help to eliminate the pathogens causing the poisoning. In the case of high fever, accompanied by other symptoms of poisoning, you should consult a physician.

• **Diarrhea and vomiting.** The diarrhea and vomiting cause the poison victim to lose a lot of liquid, putting them at risk of dehydration. To prevent this, you should try to drink liquid (water, juice, light soup) in small quantities. You should not take large quantities of liquid, since this puts the stomach walls under stress, which will cause more vomiting. If the patient suffers from diarrhea and vomiting at the same time, he should be taken immediately to the nearest doctor or emergency room.

Salmonellosis

Salmonellosis is an infection in the walls of the small intestine due to Salmonella bacteria. This infection can be caused by the ingestion of contaminated food or water. Contamination can occur during the handling and preparation of

How to find out the cause?

- To find out the origin of the poisoning, you should ask the victim the following questions:
- What have you eaten?
- How much did you eat?
- When did you eat it?
- Have you eaten anything else?
- Have you vomited?

Eggs and products made from them are closely linked to food poisoning due to *Salmonella typha*.

food if the utensils and the surrounding conditions are not sufficiently hygienic. The incubation period of salmonellosis is from 8 to 49 hours after ingestion of the contaminated food. Once the individual has been poisoned, the salmonellosis can take one or two weeks to cure. Sometimes individuals who have suffered from salmonellosis, can be carriers of the bacteria in their feces for as long as a year.

When should you suspect salmonellosis?

Salmonellosis comes from the ingestion of food in an unhealthy state, along with other factors such as:

- the ingestion of foods that are badly conserved or prepared, especially those containing eggs, chicken, and turkey.

What are the symptoms of salmonellosis?

- Muscular pain.
- Generalized pain, cramps, and abdominal pain.
- Diarrhea.
- Nausea and vomiting.
- Fever.
- Shivering.

- the keeping of pets like iguanas, tortoises, lizards and snakes, since these sometimes carry salmonella bacteria. Make sure you wash your hands thoroughly after handling such animals.

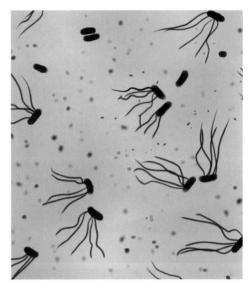

The agent causing salmonellosis is the Salmonella typha bacterium.

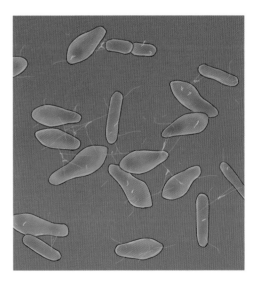

Clostridium botulinum can be found in badly preserved processed meats, home-made preserves, and some fish.

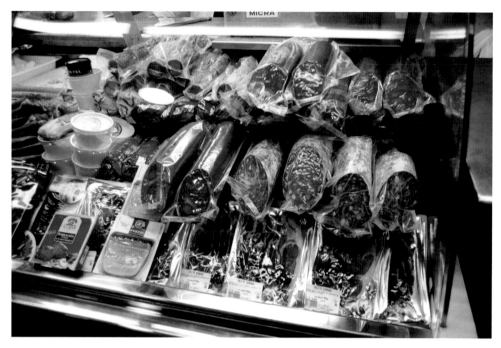

When we speak of anaerobic conditions we mean the absence of oxygen. In nature, these conditions exist at the bottom of ponds or lakes. At home, we find them mainly in canned food and airtight packages.

What should be done in a case of salmonellosis?

Most important is to maintain the level of hydration, since this is affected adversely by diarrhea. You should:

■ What are the symptoms of botulinus poisoning?

Botulinus poisoning should be suspected if canned food has been ingested on the previous day and the following symptoms are present:

- Headache
- Nausea
- Diarrhea or constipation
- Drooping eyelids
- Dry mouth
- Difficulty or inability to swallow
- Difficulty in speaking
- Difficulty in urinating

- Drink a lot of liquids.
- In case of fever or pain, take acetaminophen (Tylenol).
- Follow a strict diet (to avoid diarrhea): reduce consumption of dairy products (milk, yogurt) and have rice, apples, and bananas.

Botulinus poisoning

Botulinus poisoning (botulism) is caused by the toxins of the Clostridium botulinum bacteria. This bacillus grows in oxygen-free conditions (anaerobic), for example, in cans of meat, fish, and vegetables, and its toxin is very potent. The botulinus toxin is the most potent poison known, since one milligram is capable of killing 100 individuals. Fortunately, the toxin breaks down when heated, and is thus not found in recently cooked food.

What should be done in a case of botulinus poisoning?

If the victim has consumed canned food and has the symptoms described, he should be taken immediately to a hospital emergency room.

Mushroom poisoning

It is generally very difficult to distinguish between

Types of mushroom causing muscarinic syndrome

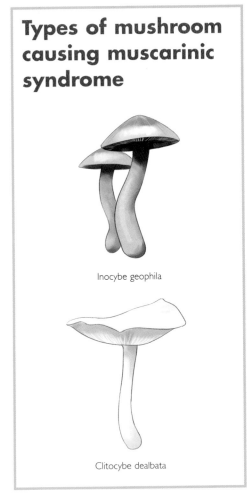

Inocybe geophila

Clitocybe dealbata

Types of mushroom causing mycoat-ropinic syndrome

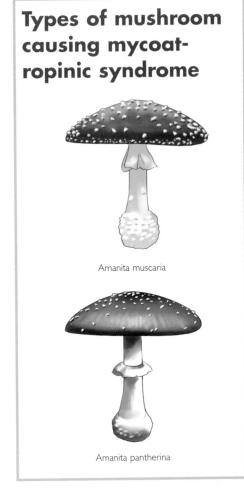

Amanita muscaria

Amanita pantherina

poisonous and non-poisonous mushrooms, since such a great variety exists. However, one can distinguish the types of poisoning according to the time it takes for the symptoms to appear. These symptoms can appear quickly or slowly.

In this kind of poisoning, the symptoms appear between half an hour and two hours after ingesting the mushroom. Among these types of poisoning, one can distinguish between the muscarinic syndrome and mycoatropinic syndrome.

The symptoms of muscarinic syndrome are the following:

- Nausea and vomiting.
- Diarrhea.
- Increase in salivation.
- Pupil contraction.
- Decreased cardiac rhythm.
- Decrease in arterial pressure.

What should you do in the case of muscarinic syndrome?

- Induce vomiting.
- Administer activated carbon (if available).
- Take the patient to hospital.

The symptoms of mycoatropinic syndrome are basically of a neurological and not gastrointestinal type, unlike the muscarinic syndrome, and are the following:

Mushroom poisoning from the *Amanita phalloides* species occurs quickly.

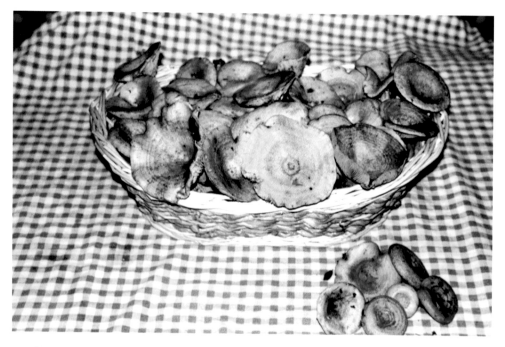

- Blurred vision.
- Dilated pupils.
- Increased cardiac rhythm.
- Confusion.
- Altered behavior.

What should you do in cases of mycoatropinic syndrome?
- Induce vomiting.
- Administer activated carbon (if available).
- Take the patient to hospital.

Poisoning with delayed appearance of symptoms
Mushroom poisoning with late appearance of symptoms can be identified when the time that elapses between the ingestion of the mushroom and the appearance of the first symptoms is greater than 6 hours, normally varying between 9 and 15 hours. In one exceptional case 15 days elapsed after ingestion of the mushroom before the first symptom. This type of poisoning is usually very serious, since the toxins damage vital organ cells.

What should you do in cases of poisoning with delayed appearance of symptoms?
In these cases, given the seriousness of this type of poisoning, priority should be given to getting the victim to hospital.

How can an edible mushroom be distinguished from a poisonous one?
Is there any way to distinguish them? There is no infallible rule for distinguishing harmless mushrooms (the great majority of those that can be found) from poisonous ones (very scarce and extremely dangerous), so that the only solution is to recognize them by their botanical features. There are many, which without being poisonous, are inedible. Their consumption should also be avoided. But you should not be too worried; with a minimum of scientific consultation, for example with a book and, preferably, with the personal help of an experienced mycologist, and remembering that, if there is any doubt about the harmlessness of a particular mushroom, the correct course is not to eat it, many scares can be avoided.

It is important to consume only those mushrooms you are familiar with and forget about the rest, both unfamiliar ones and those that are doubtful. Some of the most dangerous mushrooms have a volva, a ring, and white gills and so the most sensible thing is not to eat any with these characteristics.

Skin inflammations

Skin inflammations have many origins, given that the skin is often the first organ to come into contact with external agents or illnesses. The seriousness of the inflammations varies according to the underlying cause, although, in general, with good practical advice, they clear up quickly. It is important to keep these kinds of inflammations clean, since some of them are contagious.

General considerations and treatment at home

• Skin inflammations consist of changes in the texture or the color of the skin. These changes appear in many forms and sizes, sometimes in rings, sometimes in patches. Others can be stinging blisters, or areas of rough skin.

• Most skin inflammations are not serious and recover in a few days. However some of them require medical attention.

• Inflammation can be caused by multiple factors, such as, for example:

– Something that has come into contact with the skin, such as chemical products, latex, cosmetics, etc.

– Stress, fatigue, and extreme temperatures, which can cause seborrheic dermatitis, a type of inflammation that appears in reddish patches and skin discoloration.

– Allergies.

– Certain medicines.

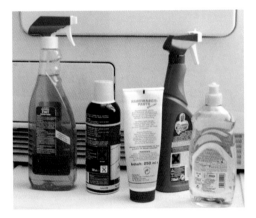

The skin is one of the first parts of the body to react when exposed to irritating substances.

– Childhood illnesses like chickenpox, measles, and rubella also cause associated skin inflammations.

Most skin inflammations can be cured using non-irritant skin products.

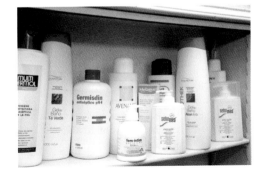

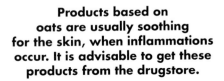

Products based on oats are usually soothing for the skin, when inflammations occur. It is advisable to get these products from the drugstore.

If the condition is extremely red, Inflamed, and very sensitive, you must go to the doctor, since any one of these symptoms might be a sign of infection.

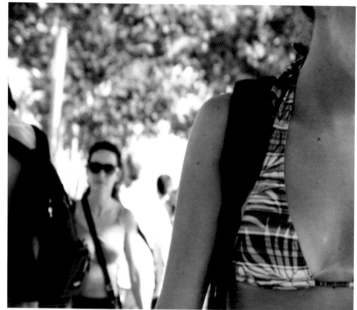

If a child suffers from measles, rubella, chickenpox, or other childhood illnesses that cause skin inflammation, you should wash your hands frequently to help prevent the spread of the micro-organism. It should never be forgotten that in any of these cases of pathology, general hygiene must be maintained rigorously.

The following general advice is recommended:
• Do not scratch or rub the skin, even if it stings.
• Try not to use soap and, where necessary, get skin-cleansing products at the drugstore.

How can you prevent skin inflammation?

• To avoid inflammations caused by typical childhood vaccines, such as those for chickenpox, measles, mumps, or rubella, you must ensure that the child follows the vaccination timetable correctly.

• If you observe that the inflammations appear after being in contact with certain substances that irritate the skin, it is better to keep away from them.

• If the inflammation is of the seborrheic dermatitis type, caused by stress, it is advisable to practice relaxation techniques like yoga, meditation or Tai Chi.

• Do not use cosmetic products on the inflammation, such as creams or skin tonics.
• During cleaning of the skin, the water should be lukewarm and the skin should be washed by patting it, without rubbing.
• As far as possible, leave the affected area in contact with the air.

When should you call the doctor in the case of a skin inflammation?
These conditions can generally be cared for at home, but you should call a doctor if the following symptoms are present:
• The sufferer's face becomes swollen.
• She has difficulty in breathing.
• She has problems swallowing, or her throat is inflamed.
• If you suspect that the inflammation is caused by a new drug prescribed by the doctor.
• If she has been stung by an insect or some other creature.
• If, after being treated at home, the inflammation is no better.

SCARLET FEVER	The child has high fever (up to 104°F (40°C), a sore throat and headache, and can also have nausea. The ganglia in the neck become inflamed and a very red rash over the whole roof of the mouth can be observed.	The rash normally appears in the groin and the armpits in the form of numerous small, soft spots in the large folds of the skin. The exanthem also covers the abdomen, chest, and back. The cheeks become flushed with fever. The chin and mouth are pale and the tongue has a very reddish color.
MEASLES	This begins with the symptoms of a very severe cold, which can last up to five days. A moderate fever, coughing, sneezing, and conjunctivitis develop. Little white spots become evident inside the mouth, surrounded by a red border. The inflammation is preceded by an abrupt rise in temperature.	First, large spots appear behind the ears, which later cover the whole face and head. They later spread to the body, arms, and legs. The spots are 3/25–1/5 inch across (35 millimeters) and in the form of slight bumps. At first, they are light red, but later they darken until they get a bluish tinge. The rash begins to disappear around the third day.
RUBELLA	This brings high fever and sweating, just like all the symptoms of a cold.	The inflammation begins behind the ears and on the face, later spreading over the whole body. The spots are bright red in color, not very big, with a slight swelling and surrounded by a light ring.
CHICKENPOX	Some 24 hours after the inflammation appears, the child loses appetite and feels a little unwell with a moderate temperature.	At first, the spots are pale red in color, but soon change into small thin blisters, surrounded by a narrow red ring. They appear especially on the back and chest, the face being hardly affected, while the feet and hands are usually free from the rash. It can also affect the mucus in the mouth. In the end, a few dry scabs remain that leave a small patch when they fall off.

Contact dermatitis

• Contact dermatitis is caused by contact with a substance that irritates the skin. The skin becomes dry and red.

• When the irritation is more severe, blisters and sores can appear on the skin.

• The substances that most frequently cause contact dermatitis are household cleaning products, such as ammonia or bleach, glues, latex, or certain plants, like nettles.

• If the person has a history of allergy, they are more likely to develop contact dermatitis.

• Sometimes, contact dermatitis can develop when the person is exposed to the substance repeatedly. At first, it does not produce irritation, but over time the person develops sensitivity to the product. This can happen with the solutions for washing contact lenses, or repeated contact with the metal of earrings.

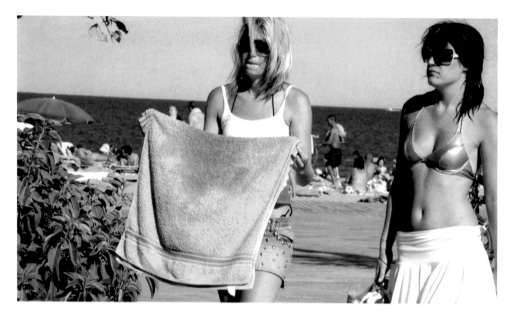

Home treatment for contact dermatitis

• First, you must clean the affected area thoroughly to get rid of any trace of the irritating substance that might have remained on the skin. If you know the substance that caused the dermatitis, it is better to avoid any contact with it.

• If the skin is inflamed, you should go to the drugstore for a corticosteroid cream. This type of cream has to be applied very carefully, since, if mis-

Some products are photosensitive, that is to say, they cause reactions only when in contact with skin that is exposed to sunlight. They are normally products for shaving, makeup, and certain perfumes. For this reason, it is advisable not to use makeup or perfume when going to the beach.

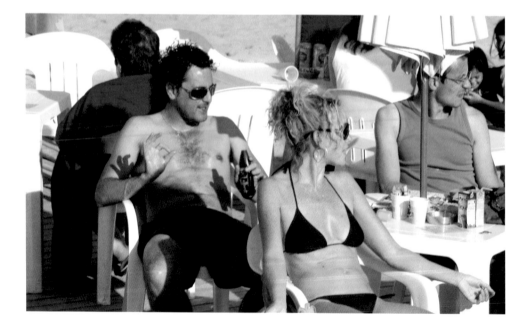

How to recognize meningitis

Meningitis is an infection of the membranes (meninges) that cover the central nervous system formed by the brain and the spinal cord. The infection can be caused by Haemophilus influenzae type b (Hib) and by Neisseria meningitidis (groups A, B, C, Y, W-135), although the most common form is viral in origin. Those affected are usually children from 3 to 8 months old, and it afflicts 1 in 100,000 people. The illness is contagious, although you have to be in close contact with the patient to get it.

Care of a meningitis patient at home

• If you suspect that anyone at home may suffer from meningitis, get immediate medical attention. People with meningitis must be hospitalized, treated with intravenous antibiotics and other medications, and their state of health should be carefully monitored.

• Once the patient has returned home, it is very important to maintain rigorous hygiene throughout the house:

The brain and spinal cord are covered by three layers of connecting tissue, which are called meninges. The nearest to the brain and spinal cord is the pia mater, the intermediate layer is called the dura mater, and the furthest from the brain and spinal cord are the arachnoids. The function of the meninges is to protect blood vessels, and to contain the cerebrospinal fluid.

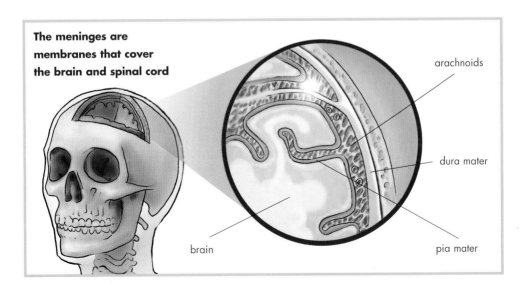

The meninges are membranes that cover the brain and spinal cord

arachnoids

dura mater

brain

pia mater

– Ensure that the person covers their mouth and nose when coughing or sneezing.

– Have minimal physical contact with the patient.

– Wash your hands frequently.

– Do not share eating utensils with the patient.

Meningitis vaccines

In most Western countries, vaccine against Haemophilus influenzae type b and meningococcal meningitis type C is recommended. This vaccine is usually administered according to the vaccination timetable for children.

In order to prevent meningitis, you should frequently check the child's vaccination record, to make sure they have received it. In case of doubt, consult the pediatrician. However, you should be aware that the vaccination against meningitis does not mean that the child is immunized against all types of meningitis.

Older children and adolescents should also be vaccinated against meningitis

What are the main symptoms of meningitis?

- Fever and shivering.
- Very intense headache.
- Nausea and vomiting.
- Stiff neck.
- Photophobia (sensitivity to light).
- Reduced consciousness.
- Neck rigidity.
- Accelerated respiration.
- Sometimes, spots on the skin.
- Kernig's or
- Brudzinski's signs of meningitis. *[See next page]*

Neisseria meningitidis

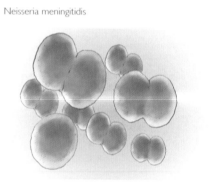

Haemophilus influenzae type b (Hib)

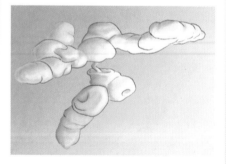

Haemophilus influenzae type b (Hib) and Neisseria meningitidis, principal pathogens causing meningitis, apart from those of viral origin.

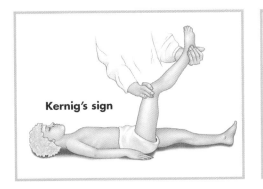

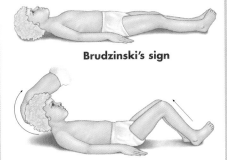

Kernig's sign is considered one of the symptoms of meningitis. If you attempt to straighten a child's leg when it is raised at an angle of 90°, and a certain rigidity in the tendons can be observed when making this movement, there is the possibility of meningitis.

Brudzinski's sign is considered another symptom of meningitis. Meningitis patients experience very severe stiffness when moving the neck, which causes the back and shoulders to bend.

The best prevention is vaccination against meningitis. However, the vaccination has some side effects.

- Inflammation in the injected area—more frequent in children of school age.
- Some fever—can occur in 5 percent of children under one and half years old.
- Irritability—frequent in children less than one year old.
- Headaches—more frequent in children over ten years old.

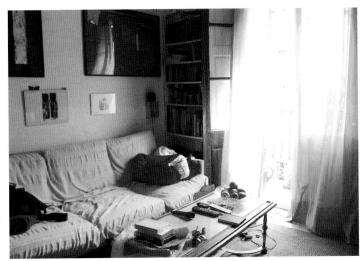

It is advisable not to share a room or remain more than five hours in a closed room with a meningitis sufferer.

Asthma attacks

When a person suffers from asthma, it is very important to know what an asthma attack is, recognize its symptoms and its warning signals so as to better control the illness, and try to stop it from interfering with everyday life.

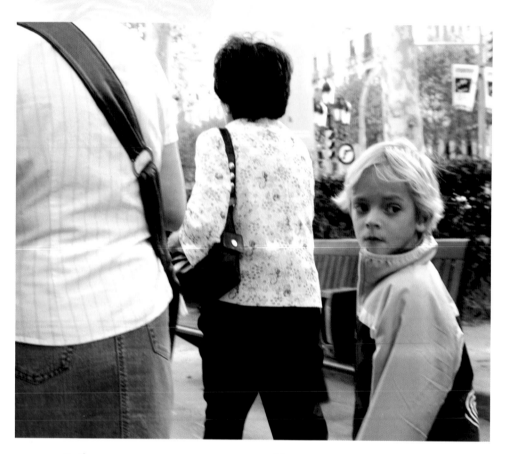

Asthma can appear at any age and is not a contagious illness. However, children who live in urban areas have more chance of contracting asthma than those in the countryside.

What is asthma?

Asthma is a chronic pulmonary illness, causing inflammation of the airways. In asthmatics, the air-ways are particularly sensitive to trigger factors, such as pollen, dust mites, tobacco fumes, or cold air. When the airways react, they become inflamed and produce more mucus than normal.

What should you do in case of an asthma attack?

- If you know what triggered the asthma attack, you must get away from it.
- Use the medication prescribed by the doctor for your asthma treatment.
- Rest for one hour until you are sure that your breathing has improved.

The reduction in airflow and the typical asthma wheezing are caused by restricted airflow in the lungs due to hardening of the muscles in the bronchial tree.

Also, the muscles surrounding the respiratory ducts contract, causing difficulty in breathing, wheezing, and a feeling of pressure in the chest. Asthma is a chronic illness that is incurable, but it can be controlled with the correct treatment.

How is asthma treated?

The object of the treatment is to control the inflammation of the airways through various types of medication:

- **Long-term control medications.** These should not be used to treat attacks; their function is to prevent them and they should be used to prolong the time between each attack. The main ones are:
  – Anti-inflammatory: Steroid inhalants.
  – Bronchodilators with prolonged action, which help to open the airways.

- **Short-term control medications.** These are used at the onset of the asthma attack. They include:
  – Short-term bronchodilators.
  – Intravenous and oral steroids. These are used in the case of a severe asthma attack. Depending on whether a person has mild or severe asthma, they are used when necessary, or

Most people are allergic to something around them, at home, at work, or at school. Avoiding these allergens can help to make asthma treatment more effective.

What are the symptoms of asthma?

- The symptoms of asthma relate to the constriction of the airways, and they include:
- Wheezing. This normally begins suddenly and usually worsens through the night or early morning. It can also get worse with exercise, or exposure to cold. The condition improves with the use of bronchodilators.
- Coughing. This may or may not be accompanied by the discharge of phlegm.
- Difficulty in breathing, which worsens with exercise or accelerated respiration.
- Difficulty in sleeping.
- Contractions of the chest muscles, that is to say, the tissue between the ribs contracts during breathing.

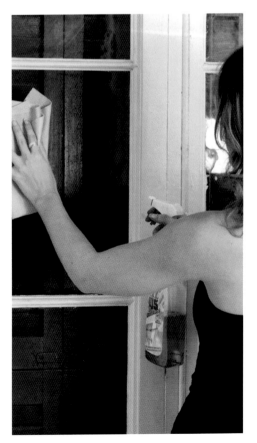

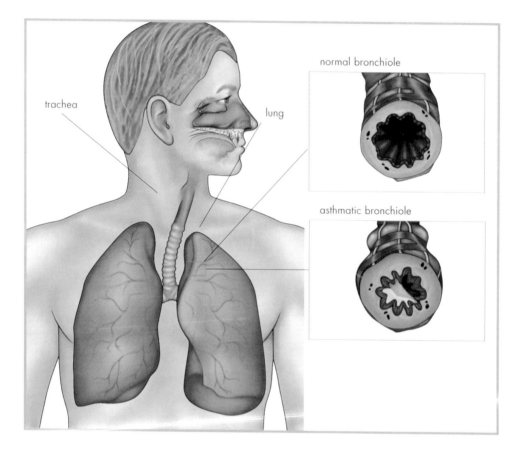

trachea

lung

normal bronchiole

asthmatic bronchiole

at regular intervals, to avoid the occurrence of attacks.

Severe asthma attacks must be controlled by a specialist, since they may require hospital admission with administration of oxygen and intravenous medication.

How can asthma attacks be prevented?

Asthma can be controlled easily if a series of steps are followed, which help prolong the interval between attacks:

• Identify the factors that trigger the attacks. Study the surroundings in which an attack occurred and look for the factors that might cause asthma. The most common factors are allergens, such as dust mites, pets, pollen, mold, some medications, and cockroaches. An asthma attack can also develop during a common cold or flu. Tobacco smoke, air fresheners, paint, hair spray, and some perfumes can also act as trigger factors. Some

The following cases require emergency treatment:

Difficulty in speaking.

When the lips or nails turn gray or bluish.
When cardiac rhythm is very accelerated.

When there is no reaction to medication.
Difficulty in walking or moving.

asthmatics also point to exercise, breathing cold air, or changes in temperature.

• Anticipation of asthma attacks. Frequently, the inflammation of airways is gradual and imperceptible. Breathing continues normally, but the scene is being set for an asthma attack. With children, it is

What is the correct way to use an inhaler?

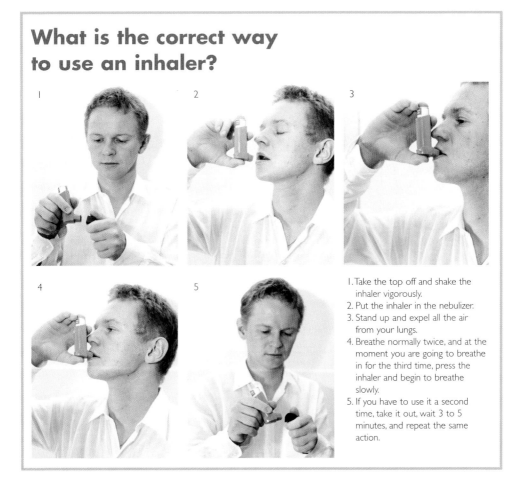

1. Take the top off and shake the inhaler vigorously.
2. Put the inhaler in the nebulizer.
3. Stand up and expel all the air from your lungs.
4. Breathe normally twice, and at the moment you are going to breathe in for the third time, press the inhaler and begin to breathe slowly.
5. If you have to use it a second time, take it out, wait 3 to 5 minutes, and repeat the same action.

helpful to notice little signs, like changes in breathing rhythm, their state of mind, or their appearance, which may indicate an impending asthma attack.

• Take the medication prescribed by the specialist. Asthma medications deal with both the symptoms and the causes, allowing them to control asthma effectively in almost any individual.

Fits of coughing

A fit of coughing causes anxiety in the sufferer. The best advice is to keep calm and not to get alarmed, breathe deeply, and swallow saliva. To soothe the throat irritation, drink water that is not very cold to hydrate yourself and even better, have a soothing hot drink with a teaspoon of honey.

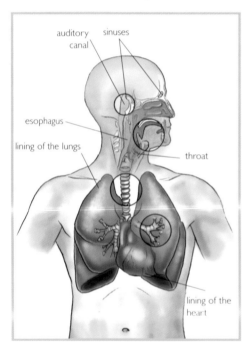

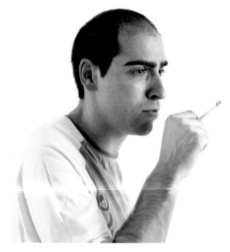

Tobacco causes chronic coughing. When you smoke and coughing attacks are happening all the time, you should consider giving up tobacco. In this is the case, you should consult a physician about the different methods of quitting.

What is coughing?

• It is a reflex action consisting of an explosive exhalation that helps to maintain the airways free of secretions and foreign bodies. It is a very frequent symptom and a common reason for consulting a specialist. However, when the coughing is excessive, it can be a sign of an underlying illness.

• A cough can be described in two ways, according to whether phlegm is produced, or according to its duration.

• In dry coughs, only air is expelled; in expellant coughs, there is expectoration (sputum).

• Severe coughs are characterized by a sudden onset, being generally caused by colds, flu, or infection in the upper respiratory tracts. A "chronic cough" is when it lasts more than two weeks; this is usually due to tobacco or certain allergies.

Coughing is a defense mechanism; coughing protects the airways and keeps them clean for breathing.

◾ What are the causes of coughing?

If you suffer a severe fit of coughing, it is advisable to take cough medication in the form of tablets or syrup.

The causes of coughing are very diverse and among them the following are significant:

- Chills, colds, and flu.
- Nose, ear, and throat ailments.
- Pulmonary infections, such as pneumonia and acute bronchitis.
- Chronic pulmonary illnesses, such as asthma and chronic bronchitis.
- Illnesses of the external auditory duct.
- Gastro-esophageal reflux.
- Accidental causes, for example, the entry of foreign bodies into the trachea, smoke, etc.

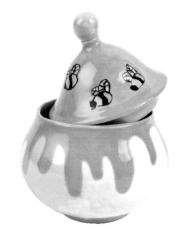

Advice for smoking mothers

It is scientifically proven that nicotine finds its way into mother's milk, although the levels are not harmful for the baby. It is therefore advisable to breastfeed a baby even if the mother is a smoker.

- Smoking mothers are advised to quit tobacco, but, if they are unable to give up the habit, they can follow a series of recommendations:
- Do not smoke in the house, or in the baby's room.
- Try to cut down on cigarettes.
- Continue breastfeeding, bearing in mind the protection it offers against infections caused by tobacco.
- After smoking, allow at least two hours before breastfeeding. Although the nicotine levels may not be toxic for babies, they can still cause a number of unpleasant effects.
- Nicotine has a stimulating effect, so that babies of smoking mothers will be less inclined to sleep and rest than babies of non-smoking mothers.
- Babies of smokers have a greater propensity to suffer from cot death syndrome.

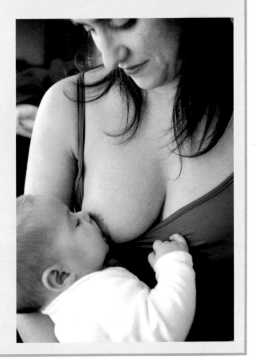

What should you do in the event of a coughing fit?

- Coughing fits cause anxiety in the sufferer. First, try to relax the individual having the fit and advise him to breathe deeply and swallow saliva.

- If there is stinging in the throat, cough drops or candies can be taken, but they should not be given to children under three for risk of choking. They should contain honey and herbs for soothing the throat; however, menthol should be avoided, because it produces irritation.

- If the cause of the cough is a chill, mucus will slide from the nose down to the throat, provoking a cough. This situation gets worse at night when you are lying in bed; it is therefore advisable to sleep with your head slightly higher, adding additional pillows.

- You should drink a lot of liquid to dilute the mucus and ease its expulsion.

- In order to alleviate inflammation in the throat, have a hot drink with honey, or a glass of water that is not too cold.

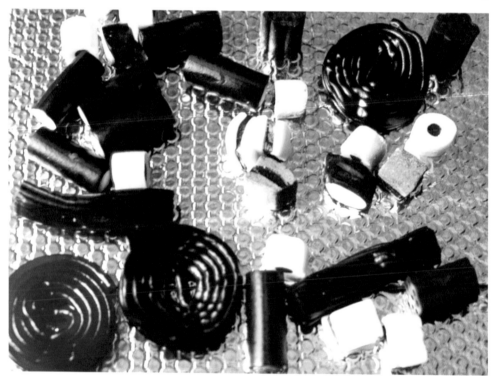

Licorice has anti-coughing and expectorant properties. It helps to calm coughing and to reduce irritation of the airways. It can be taken, always in moderation, in the form of infusion, candy, or by chewing a licorice stick.

One of the most common causes of chronic coughing is bronchitis. This is characterized by inflammation of the bronchial tubes, which produces coughing with sputum. Among the causes of this illness are tobacco, pollution, infection of the airways, and allergies.

Fits and convulsions

Fits or convulsions can be dangerous for the sufferer because of the injuries that can be sustained. Convulsions can be the result of very high fever, illnesses such as epilepsy, drug taking, or blows to the head.

What is epilepsy?

This is a condition of the central nervous system, caused by increased neuronal activity in the brain. It affects all ages, although it occurs most frequently in childhood, adolescence, and old age. In developing countries, its occurrence can be due to obstetric problems and infections of the central nervous system.

For a person to be considered epileptic, the fits must occur with a certain frequency. Children may present very similar symptoms to those of epilepsy, including convulsions, when they have very high fever, or receive a hard blow to the head.

What are the symptoms of epilepsy?

Epilepsy attacks are of two main types. In attacks known as the grand mal, the person falls to the ground, becomes rigid and begins to have convulsions. In the other type of attack, known as the petit mal, the person remains with a fixed stare for a few seconds. In other types of attack, the person acts as though half-awake, or makes abrupt limb movements, or experiences changes in perception of his surroundings.

The alarm signals that warn of an impending epilepsy attack are:
• Mental confusion.
• Appearance of involuntary movements in the jaws or eyes.
• A feeling of extreme fatigue.
• Inability to maintain a conversation or respond to simple question.
• Finally, the appearance of convulsions.

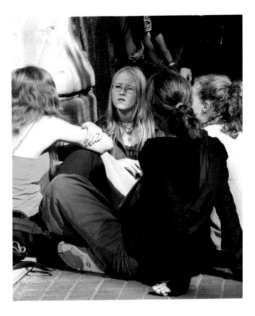

At present, epilepsy is one of the most common cerebral illnesses. Studies conducted by the World Health Organization and International Bureau for Epilepsy estimate that 1–2 percent of the population suffer from this condition, the most affected being children, adolescents under 20 years old, and the elderly. One of the main problems faced by epilepsy sufferers stems from the ignorance that exists in society regarding this affliction. It is a poorly understood illness that arouses fear, secrecy, and even the marginalizing of those who suffer from it. It should not be forgotten that epilepsy is a noncontagious neurological illness, not a mental illness, nor a cause of backwardness.

What should you do in the case of a fit of epilepsy?

• Remain calm and make sure that other people around the sufferer do likewise.

• Lay the person on the ground, to prevent him falling and injuring himself.

• If you know the sufferer and they have said that they have the anti-epileptic medication, put the medication in their mouth just before the convulsions occur or just afterwards. Trying to make them take it during the convulsions is useless, because the digestive system ceases to function during a fit.

• In the course of the convulsions, avoid being hit by a blow from the person, since they can sometimes hit very hard.

• Move objects away from the sufferer to prevent them injuring themselves with something.

• During the attack, uncontrolled movements of the mouth and tongue are a normal occurrence. To avoid possible injuries, a long hard object should be placed in the sufferer's mouth.

• Place a pillow under the head, or some article of clothing folded double, to prevent him hitting his head on the ground.

• Once the attack is over, the sufferer should not be left alone, as he will feel very confused and probably will not remember where he is or what has happened.

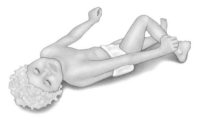

During febrile convulsions, a child flexes and extends his limbs.

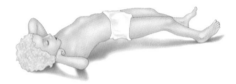

What not to do

• Do not give artificial respiration.

• Do not shake or hit the sufferer. You should wait patiently for the fit to pass.

• Do not apply alcohol to their forehead.

• Do not try to make the sufferer swallow anti-epileptic medication during the attack, since the swallowing mechanism does not function during the fit.

When to call the doctor or an ambulance

• If the convulsions last more than five minutes.

• If the sufferer is diabetic or pregnant.

What are the signs of febrile convulsions?

High fever usually precedes this type of convulsion. The other symptoms include:

• Loss of consciousness.

• Grand mal type of convulsions or tonic-clonic seizure.

• Violent movement of the limbs and face.

• Difficulty in breathing.

• On regaining consciousness, the child is irritable.

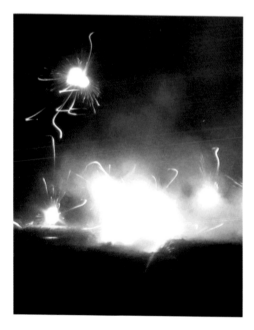

In most cases, the cause of epilepsy attacks is unpredictable, but sometimes very bright or flashing lights can trigger an attack.

What are febrile convulsions?

On the majority of occasions when a child has convulsions, this is due to fever, which is why they are called febrile convulsions.

During these, children often lose consciousness and shake.

Most episodes last 1–2 minutes.

The fact that a child is prone to suffering febrile convulsions does not mean that he is more likely to suffer from epilepsy, since epileptic convulsions are not caused by fever.

This type of convulsion affects 1 to 5 percent of the infant population, and there is a genetic predisposition to suffer from them.

The majority of febrile convulsions occur during the first day of the child's fever.

What should you do if your child has febrile convulsions?

• Try to turn him on his side to prevent choking.

• Leave him asleep, away from objects that might injure him.

If the child vomits, lay him on his side. This prevents vomit entering the lungs .

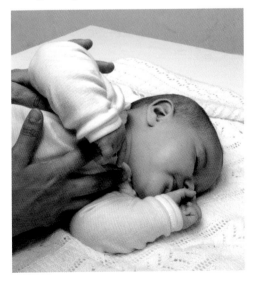

• Do not get hold of the child during the convulsion.

• Remain calm and wait for the convulsion to pass.

• Put a cushion under his head.

• Loosen any clothing that might constrain him.

• Do not put anything in his mouth.

• Call the emergency medical services if the convulsion lasts more than 10 minutes.

• When the convulsions are over, try to reduce the fever, for example with acetaminophen (Tylenol), and applying cool cloths to the forehead.

▪ What to do in the event of a fit or convulsion (non-epileptic)

• Above all, remain calm at all times.

• Do not try to restrain the body movements of the sufferer, or hold him closely, or lift him up during the fit or convulsion.

• Remove furniture and objects near the sufferer, to prevent self-harm.

• Loosen clothing, to facilitate breathing.

• Do not give anything to eat or drink.

• When the convulsion or attack is over, place the person on his left side with his head on a pillow. Talk to him softly and affectionately so that he can gradually come round.

• If breathing stops, give artificial respiration while the emergency medical services are on their way.

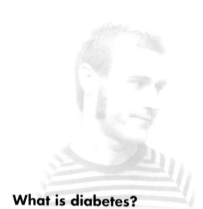

Emergencies with diabetics

Diabetes sufferers may experience one or more of the emergency situations characteristic of the disease, such as insulin reaction or diabetic coma.

What is diabetes?

Diabetes is a chronic illness, which is characterized by the presence of high levels of sugar in the blood. The cause is usually the under-production of insulin by the pancreas, the resistance of the organism to insulin, or both factors at the same time.

There are three main types of diabetes:

• **Type 1.** This occurs when the pancreas produces very little or no insulin. To survive, it is necessary to take insulin daily (generally in the form of injections).

• **Type 2.** Approximately 90 percent of diabetes diagnosed belongs to this category. It appears in adult life and comes from the pancreas's inability to produce sufficient insulin to maintain normal levels of glucose in the blood. This type of diabetes is increasing in Western populations, due to obesity and lack of exercise.

• **Gestational.** During pregnancy, a non-diabetic woman can have abnormally high levels of glucose.

How can diabetes be controlled?

Diabetes is controlled by maintaining the levels of glucose in the blood at normal values (70–110 mg/dL). This can be achieved both through fasting and diet regulation. Control is managed by balancing three principal elements:

• Treatment. Depending on the type of diabetes, insulin is taken in the form of injections or oral medication.

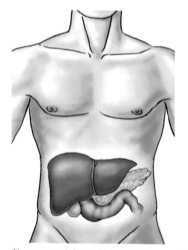

The pancreas is located behind the liver and is the organ where insulin is produced. Insulin is the hormone regulating the use and storage of glucose.

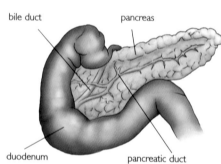

bile duct   pancreas

duodenum   pancreatic duct

Insulin is a hormone produced by the pancreas, whose function is to regulate the levels of sugar in the blood.

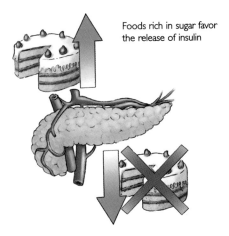

Foods rich in sugar favor the release of insulin

Understanding how the pancreas functions and releases insulin helps a diabetic to control the levels of glucose through diet.

• Dietary control. Food raises levels of sugar, and exercise and insulin lowers them. Diabetics should know when and what to eat.

• An exercise program. Diabetics are strongly recommended to take exercise in order to maintain the levels of glucose within the normal range.

Insulin reaction or hypoglycemia

Diabetics who require insulin or medications that lower the level of sugar can sometimes suffer a reduction in sugar below normal levels, causing hypoglycemia.

Hypoglycemia is not usually serious, although it is necessary to be very familiar with its symptoms to be able to treat it in time, because if not, it can become dangerous.

If a glucose measuring kit is not available and the symptoms of hypoglycemia are present, the individual should have something sweet anyway. You should wait for 15 minutes, for sugar levels to return to normal. If the symptoms have disappeared after 15 minutes, some food should then be eaten, not when the symptoms are first evident, since in order to make them go away, simple sugars should be consumed and not more complex food.

If, after 15 minutes, the symptoms do not improve or get worse, you should ask the diabetic if he has glucagon injections so that he can be given one. If he does not, he should go to the emergency room immediately.

What are the symptoms of hypoglycemia?

• Occurs suddenly.
• Attention lapses and confusion.
• Pale complexion.
• Drowsiness.
• Inappropriate responses.
• Headache.
• Sudden hunger.
• Lack of coordination.
• Sickness.
• Trembling.
• Sweating.
• Bad temper.
• Blurred vision.

▪ What should you do in the case of hypoglycemia?

If the diabetic has a glucose measuring kit, you should test the level of sugar in his blood. If the relevant level is below 70 mg/dL, he should have some food with a high sugar content such as:

• Fruit juice.

• A soft drink.

• Something sweet.

Hyperglycemia

In contrast to hypoglycemia, hyperglycemia consists in the abnormal increase in levels of sugar in the blood (70 to 110 mg/dL). If the level rises above 180 mg/dL, this indicates hyperglycemia. If this level continues increasing up to levels of 240 mg/dL, the patient may fall into a diabetic coma, a very dangerous situation. This usually occurs in individuals who do not follow their treatment correctly. It is proven that high levels of sugar are related to a greater risk of infections and complications in the long term.

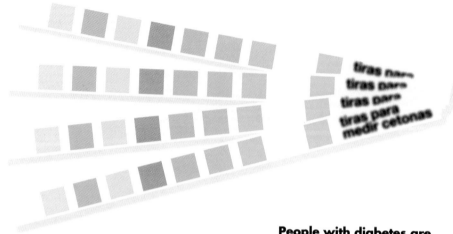

People with diabetes are recommended to have ketone measuring strips at their disposal, so as to control ketone levels in case of hyperglycemia. The presence of ketones in the blood during hyperglycemia is very serious and may lead to coma.

What should you do in the case of hyperglycemia?

- First, if the diabetic shows symptoms of hyperglycemia and has a glucose measuring kit, his level should be tested.
- If there are ketones in your urine, you should go to the doctor immediately.
- If there are no ketones, it is advisable to go back to your usual treatment for diabetes so that normal levels of glucose in the blood can be restored.
- If the levels do not fall, consult your doctor.

What are ketones?

Ketones are substances that accumulate in the blood when fats break down, and they appear when there are imbalances in the levels of insulin in the blood.

What are the symptoms of hyperglycemia?

- In contrast to the symptoms of hypoglycemia, those of hyperglycemia appear gradually.
- Extraordinary thirst and a very dry mouth.
- Urge to urinate too frequently.
- Lethargy and drowsiness.
- Fatigue and exhaustion.
- Breath smelling of fruit.
- Wounds slow to form scabs.

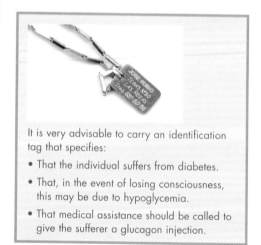

It is very advisable to carry an identification tag that specifies:

- That the individual suffers from diabetes.
- That, in the event of losing consciousness, this may be due to hypoglycemia.
- That medical assistance should be called to give the sufferer a glucagon injection.

Blackouts, fainting, and loss of consciousness

Blackouts, fainting, and loss of consciousness are normally momentary events. They may be a symptom of an underlying pathology, for example heart disease, or they may appear by themselves due to some powerful emotion. In general, they do not lead to complications and disappear in a few minutes. But if they are recurrent, you should consult a physician to find out their cause.

What are blackouts, fainting, and loss of consciousness?

Blackouts, also known as loss of consciousness or fainting, consist in passing out for a brief period of time, normally less than two minutes. This occurs when not enough blood reaches the brain.

The individuals affected usually complain of vertigo and sickness before fainting. When the loss of consciousness is more prolonged, it is called coma. It is estimated that more than half the population

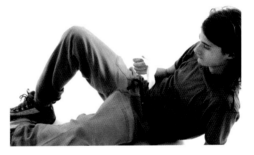

In general, recovery from fainting fits is swift and complete; the sufferer recovers in a few minutes.

What are the causes of blackouts, fainting, and loss of consciousness?

In 95 percent of cases, there is no clear cause of fainting, if there are no underlying illnesses present. The remaining 5 percent of cases are caused by cardiac disease.

The most common factors are:

- Fear.
- Pain.
- Stress.
- Heat.
- Exhaustion.

have suffered a fainting fit at some moment in their lives.

- Fainting usually occurs when an individual is standing or sitting, very rarely in cases where the person is lying down, although it can occur when a person tries to get up abruptly.
- If the fainting occurs when your head is moved to one side, this could mean that the neck bones are interrupting the flow of blood from the arteries up to the brain. When this occurs, call a doctor.
- A fall in blood sugar levels can also cause fainting, which usually occurs in diabetic patients, although it also occurs in individuals who haven't had food for a long period.
- Women with low blood pressure are more prone to suffer from fainting.

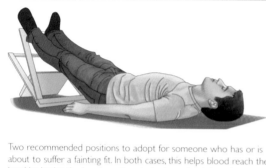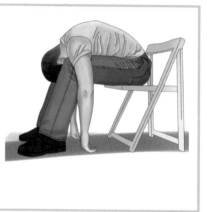

Two recommended positions to adopt for someone who has or is about to suffer a fainting fit. In both cases, this helps blood reach the head by having the head positioned at a lower level than the rest of the body.

• Other more serious problems, such as heart disease or epileptic fits, can cause fainting.

• Some medications can also cause fainting as a side effect. You should consult your doctor if you suspect that such losses of consciousness relate to a medication you are taking.

• More rarely, you can suffer a fainting fit when urinating or coughing, since this can interrupt blood supply to the brain. It is advisable to consult a doctor if it is a situation that recurs more than once.

• The consumption of alcohol and drugs such as cocaine or marijuana can also cause lapses in consciousness.

What to look out for in cases of blackouts, fainting, and loss of consciousness

The main signs that someone is going to faint are the following:

• The individual feels suddenly weak and sick.

• If he is sitting, he feels he is going to fall off the seat or the bed.

• He can also feel queasiness in his stomach.

• Pale appearance.

• Cold sweats.

• Blurred vision.

• Loss of consciousness.

• Shallow breathing.

• Weak pulse.

• Falling to the ground.

What should be done in the case of fainting?

• If you observe that an individual is about to faint, you should try to make him sit or lie down.

• When someone feels he is about to faint, he should immediately warn those near him and go to a chair or bed, and try not to knock against anything around him.

• Loosen the clothing of someone who has suffered a fainting fit.

• Move the head to one side, to avoid suffocation or choking in case of vomiting.

• Raise the person's feet about a foot (30 cm) above the level of his heart.

• The individual should remain lying down at least 10 minutes, in a peaceful cool place. If the windows are closed, open them. He should avoid direct sunlight.

• If there is no suitable place for the person to stretch out, he should be made to lean forward with his head placed between his knees, or level with his abdomen or waist.

• Do not try to give liquids or solids until he has completely recovered consciousness.

• Examine the airways, opening his mouth in search of objects that might be obstructing the breathing.

• Take his pulse.

• If necessary, do cardiopulmonary resuscitation.

When should you call a doctor in case of blackouts, fainting, and loss of consciousness?

• If the individual who has fainted is apparently healthy and has only fainted on this one occasion, there is no reason to worry and no need to call a doctor, since fainting is fairly common and recovery is total without the need for treatment.

• If the individual who has fainted suffers from cardiac disease, has high blood pressure, or is diabetic, it is advisable to see a doctor.

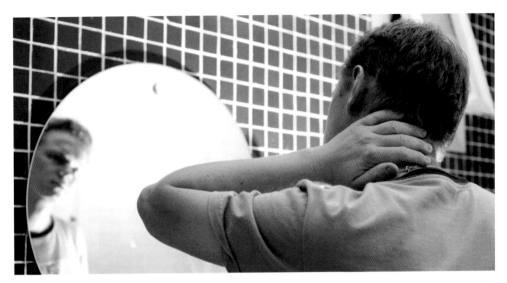

Individuals with neck problems also suffer from fainting, although this is usually accompanied by other symptoms of lack of blood supply to the brain, such as vertigo or inability to maintain posture.

Call a doctor if the fainting is accompanied by the following additional symptoms:

– The individual does not regain consciousness after two minutes.

– It is a pregnant woman who has fainted.

– If the sufferer is an individual over 50 years old.

– The person who has fainted has diabetes (in that case, check if they have a medical identification bracelet).

– The presence of chest pain.

– Irregular heartbeat.

– Difficulty in breathing.

– The fainting occurs suddenly without any previous discomfort or sickness.

– The person affected is confused.

– Blurred vision.

– Difficulty in speaking.

– The individual faints when turning his head to one side.

– When the sufferer faints more than once a month.

– In elderly people, if the fainting recurs frequently or normally happens after physical effort.

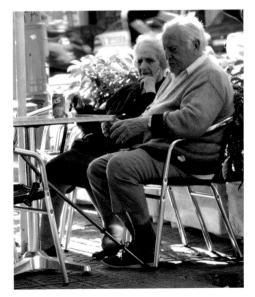

You should call a doctor in cases where the individual who has fainted has been injured on falling to the ground, especially with elderly people, since this can cause a bone fracture.

Cardiac arrest (heart failure)

Cardiac arrests are the cause of urgent admissions to hospitals, and if not treated in time, may be fatal. It is thus very important to recognize the symptoms associated with this emergency and to follow a series of instructions for keeping the casualty alive, while waiting for the arrival of the emergency medical services.

What is a cardiac arrest?

The heart pumps blood to the rest of the body in two phases: systolic and diastolic.

• **Diastole.**

First, the blood accumulates in the upper chambers of the heart (right and left auricles). The heart muscle has a natural pacemaker that, at a certain moment, triggers the contraction of the auricles. When these contract, the blood passes through the tricuspid and mitral valves into the right and left ventricles.

• **Systole.**

This second phase begins when the ventricles are full of blood. The natural pacemaker gives the signal for the ventricles to contract. In order to prevent blood returning to the auricles, the tricuspid and mitral valves close and the pulmonary and aortic valves open.

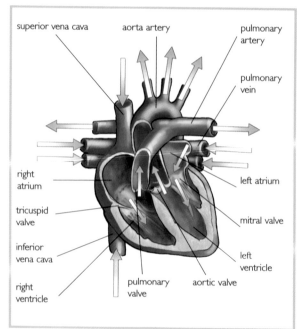

superior vena cava   aorta artery   pulmonary artery

pulmonary vein

right atrium

left atrium

tricuspid valve

mitral valve

inferior vena cava

left ventricle

right ventricle

pulmonary valve   aortic valve

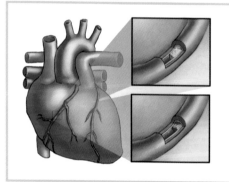

The cause of cardiac arrest is the formation of a clot or spasm in one of the arteries that supply oxygen to the cardiac muscle, causing damage to the coronary tissue.

• This allows the right ventricle to push the blood towards the lungs to oxygenate it, while oxygenated blood leaves the left ventricle to circulate the body.

• When the blood has passed through the lungs and the rest of the body, the ventricles relax, and

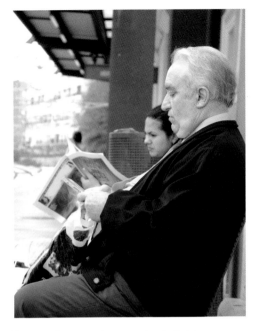

Heart attacks are not always associated with intense chest pain. In women and elderly people, the symptoms may possibly be less severe.

the tricuspid and mitral valves open again, beginning the cycle once more.

• The brain detects the external conditions (such as exercise, stress, and climate) and regulates the heart rhythm.

• When the heart stops beating, this is a cardiac arrest.

What are the causes of cardiac arrest?

Most heart attacks are due to coronary diseases, although other less common causes exist:

• Suffocation
• Hypothermia
• Severe blows to the head.
• Electrocution.
• Very severe hemorrhages, which may be internal, caused by a blow, or external, such as those caused by a sharp weapon.
• Severe dehydration, like that caused by cholera, associated with very severe diarrhea.
• Inhalation of toxic gases, such as smoke from a fire or carbon monoxide, like that expelled by certain heating systems that malfunction.
• Very severe asthma attacks.
• Strangulation.

The most usual medication in the case of heart attacks is nitroglycerin in the form of tablets, which are placed under the tongue.

• Very severe allergic reaction (anaphylactic shock).
• Drug overdoses.
• Poisoning.

What are the symptoms of cardiac arrest?

You should suspect that someone is suffering a cardiac arrest if he has the following symptoms:

• Sudden loss of consciousness.
• Not responding to gentle shaking.
• Abnormal or interrupted breathing.
• They do not move or cough.

If the cause of cardiac arrest is a heart attack, the symptoms are as follows:

• Chest pain, under the sternum, which can spread out to the arms, neck, or abdomen.
• Pain in the face, teeth, and jaw.
• More subtle pains, like feelings of compression.
• Sudden failure in respiration.
• Sickness, vertigo, and vomiting.

In the case of children:

• Loss of consciousness.
• Their skin can turn blue.

Should you always call the emergency medical services?

When dealing with a life-threatening emergency, you must contact the emergency medical services immediately if:

• The chest pain is sudden and accompanied by the other heart attack symptoms.

• The person is unconscious and has stopped breathing.

• After carrying out cardiopulmonary resuscitation for 1 minute—or immediately if you do not know the resuscitation techniques.

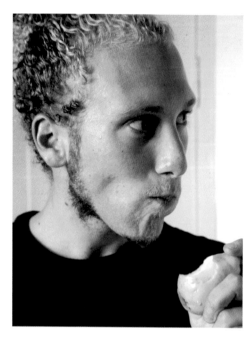

Maintaining a healthy diet from childhood helps to reduce the risk of coronary diseases in adult life.

tation is not carried out, the patient may die in a few minutes. It is therefore advisable to do the following:

– Make the patient sit down and be comfortable. He should remain as relaxed as possible.

– Loosen any clothing that might constrict.

– Ask the patient if he suffers from any heart disease and if so, whether he has his medication with him; if that is the case, help him to take it.

– If the pain does not stop after 3 minutes, call the emergency medical services.

If the patient is unconscious:

– Begin cardiorespiratory resuscitation procedures.

– Call the emergency medical services.

If the patient is a baby or a child who is unconscious:

– Begin cardiorespiratory resuscitation procedures.

– Call the emergency medical services.

What should you do in the case of cardiac arrest?

This type of emergency is not followed by the victim's spontaneous recovery and if cardiac resusci-

Sudden infant death syndrome consists of the sudden death of a healthy child less than one year old without apparent cause.

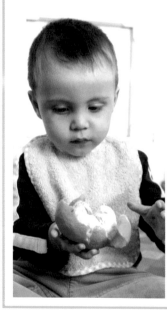

Cardiac arrest in children

• Cardiac arrest in children can be caused by congenital coronary diseases, although in the majority of cases, it is the result of an earlier respiratory failure, whose causes may be:

– Accidental ingestion of foreign bodies.

– Smoke inhalation.

– Suffocation.

– Sudden infant death syndrome.

• You MUST carry out cardiopulmonary resuscitation procedures and call the emergency medical services immediately if the child:

– does not respond to stimuli,

– is not breathing,

– has an imperceptible pulse and is very weak,

– and has turned pale and bluish in his skin.

Panic and anxiety attacks

Anxiety keeps you alert in threatening situations. But anxiety can often overwhelm and become uncontrollable, causing a negative effect, meaning a breakdown in the most serious cases.

What is a panic attack and how does it manifest itself?

• A panic attack consists of an experience of extreme anxiety, accompanied by intense fear and unease. Such attacks usually occur abruptly and reach their maximum intensity in the first 10 minutes.

• It is thought that panic attacks occur more frequently in women than men. Generally, children do not suffer this type of episode; it normally occurs from around the age of 25.

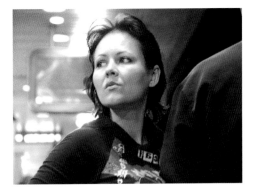

A panic attack is an experience of anxiety that may be associated with agoraphobia: the fear of public places and situations beyond our control.

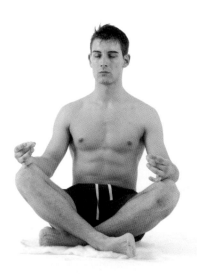

• Individuals who have suffered a panic attack continue to fear that they will suffer another one in the months following.

• Panic attacks are normally associated with the following symptoms:
  – Palpitations.
  – Increased heart rate.
  – Sweating.
  – Trembling and shaking.

When an individual feels his anxiety increasing, he should try to breathe regularly and relax when he exhales.

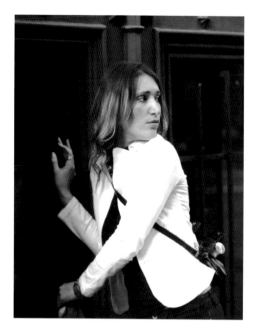

If excessive worry and nervousness are almost daily events, and last for at least six months, the condition can be described as "anxiety disorder." This is chronic tension with no apparent cause. It can sometimes be associated with depression.

– Sensation of suffocation or lack of breath.
– Sensation of choking.
– Pressure or discomfort in the chest.
– Nausea and abdominal discomfort.
– Lack of balance.
– Sickness or feeling faint.
– Sensation of numbness and anxiety.
– Shivering or suffocation.
– Strange, altered perception of self and surroundings.
– Fear of death, going mad, or losing control.

What should you do in the case of a panic attack?

Individuals who suffer panic attacks must normally be treated by a specialist. It has been demonstrated that a combination of drugs and psychotherapy helps to reduce the frequency of this type of attack.

However, if they do occur, certain steps may be followed in order to control them:
• Try to be aware that the feelings of fear and insecurity are only exaggerated normal reactions to a stressful situation.

• Explain to the sufferer of an attack that what he is feeling is only sensations, not reality. If during the attack, the person thinks he is going to die or is very ill, remind him that although he feels this, it is completely untrue.
• Tell the sufferer not to struggle against these sensations, but to let them pass in the same way that they appeared.
• Find a quiet place, where the person can relax. If he is on the street, he should lean on something or sit down.
• The person should concentrate on what is happening at that moment, not what might happen.
• When the fear diminishes, he should breathe deeply and continue his activities.

Anxiety

• In normal situations, nervousness and tension in response to a stimulus provide a level of caution and help to maintain concentration to confront the challenge that is causing the anxiety. Furthermore, everybody has felt anxiety at some point in their lives—for example nervousness before an exam, tension at work and a sick feeling in the stomach before a particular appointment. However, this same tension, if it becomes exaggerated, can produce undesired effects, preventing you from facing up to situations. Under

The main symptoms of anxiety are:

• Extreme nervousness, disquiet, or impatience.
• Tiredness and fatigue.
• Difficulty in concentrating.
• Irritability.
• Muscular tension, trembling, headaches, leg movements, and inability to relax.
• Alterations in sleeping pattern: difficulty getting to sleep or remaining asleep or sensation of waking up unrefreshed.
• Sweating, palpitations, or tachycardia, gastrointestinal problems, dry mouth, sickness, hyperventilation (increase in the number of breaths per minute).

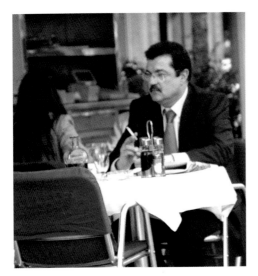

If the anxiety disorder originates from work, the sufferer must learn to balance his responsibilities with recreation.

such circumstances,we speak of an anxiety attack.

• Anxiety attacks can occur with different intensity and in different forms. The way that anxiety is expressed is also different in each individual. There are people who experience anxiety at very specific moments in their lives, for example before an exam. In others, it can be felt throughout the day, making them excessively worried, whether about their family, money, or health.

What should you do in the case of anxiety?

• Anxiety attacks should be treated by a specialist. The treatment usually consists of a combination of psychotherapy, drugs, and relaxation techniques.

• Also, changes in lifestyle can be put into practice, which help the individual with an anxiety disorder to feel more relaxed:

– Control sleep patterns. Sleep the necessary amount, get up and go to bed each day at the same time.

– Take moderate exercise.

– Reduce consumption of alcohol and tobacco.

– Follow a healthy and balanced diet.

– Do not take drugs.

– Learn relaxation techniques—yoga, tai chi, and meditation are helpful in the case of anxiety.

– Do handicrafts, painting, or play a musical instrument.

Nightmares in children

Most children have a nightmare once in a while and one in four have nightmares more than once a week. Generally, they begin at the age of two, although they are more common at three to six years of age. The majority of nightmares occur between four and six in the morning and can repeat several nights in succession. The most common causes are:

• Anxiety and stress (responsible for more than half of cases).

• Illness with fever.

• Death of a loved one.

• Side effects of medications.

What should be done in case of nightmares?

The main advice to follow is try to calm the child down, keep her company, and give her your attention:

• Try to prevent the nightmares, by supervising the television programs that the child watches, especially if she watches them before going to bed.

• After a nightmare, do not leave the child alone until she feels completely at ease, even though you run the risk of losing sleep. Sometimes, reading a book with the child or telling a story or a little tale helps her to calm down.

• Relax the child talking to them in a calm gentle voice.

• If the child is old enough to talk, you should try to encourage her to talk about her nightmare and invent a happy ending to it. If the child prefers not to talk about the dream, do not insist.

• Do not wake the child if she is crying in her sleep and not too upset. The most likely thing is that the nightmare will pass and the child will sleep peacefully afterward.

It is not a good practice to allow children to sleep with their parents after a nightmare, since, besides making them afraid of their own bed, it may become a habit.

Foreign bodies in the eyes or ears

A foreign body is some element alien to the organism, which enters it, perhaps through the skin or some natural orifice, such as the eyes, nose, or throat, impeding its normal functioning.

Foreign bodies in the eyes

• Examples of foreign bodies in the eye are badly placed contact lenses, particles of sand or metal, makeup, eyelashes and insects, etc.

• They can lodge under the eyelid as well as the eyeball.

• It is necessary to take out these foreign bodies as soon as possible, since they can have irritating effects, cause scratches to the eye or penetrate it.

• When a foreign body enters the eye, it provokes the following symptoms:

– Inflammation of the eyelid.

– Reddening of the affected eye.

– Burning sensation.

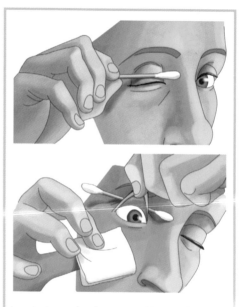

In order to examine the upper eyelid, take a Q-Tip and place it over the lid. Then pull the eyelid gently upward so that you can see behind it. If you have to cover it or manipulate it further, use sterile gauze.

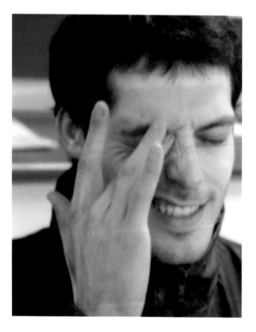

– Pain.

– Tears.

– Difficulty in keeping the eye open.

The eye is a very delicate area in the body that can easily be injured. It is necessary to treat any damage that can occur to it immediately, since otherwise you may lose your sight.

How to bandage an eye

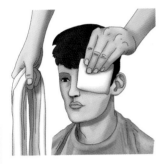 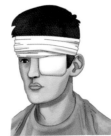 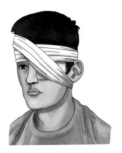 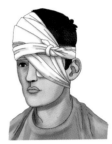

1. Protect the eye with sterile gauze.

2. Wind the bandage twice around the head at forehead level securing the upper edge of the sterile gauze.

3. Wind the the bandage lower down, over the affected eye, covering it and pass the bandage under the ear on the same side.

4. Repeat the operation until the eye is completely covered.

What should be done in the case of a foreign body entering the eye?

If it is a small object under the eyelid:

• Wash your hands with soap and water before examining the injured eye.

• Try not to rub your eye.

• Examine the affected eye with a lamp or flashlight so that you can see it clearly. Ask the individual to sit down, with his head tilted back, so that the light points directly into the injured eye.

• In order to locate the foreign body, the individual must first look up and down and then from left to right. If the foreign body cannot be found, gently lift the lower eyelid to see whether it is there. If it is, ask the individual to look up and then carefully remove the object. If it is not there, do the same with the upper eyelid. To do this, you can use a Q-Tip, placing it on the upper eyelid and rolling the eyelid back gently.

• If the foreign body is inside the eyelid, it should be washed out with plenty of water. If the object does not come out, a second Q-Tip can be used to gently remove it.

• If the object is embedded in the eye, you should cover the eye with sterile gauze, bandage it, and go to the doctor. Do not take out the foreign body or use eye drops.

Foreign bodies in the ears

• Children often put objects in their ears, which are difficult to extract. Given that the auditory duct has very thin skin, any element that presses on the skin there causes very severe pain.

• It is necessary to take out any foreign body that has entered the ear immediately, since this will considerably decrease the danger of infection.

• When an object has been placed in the ear, the following symptoms are common:

– Pain and inflammation.

– If the foreign object is an insect, you may feel it moving inside the ear.

– Hearing may be reduced.

– Nausea and vomiting.

– Bleeding from the ear.

What should be done in the case of a foreign body in the ear?

• If it is an object:

– Try to calm the individual.

– If the object is visible and protruding, take it out carefully with some tweezers. Then call the doctor to make sure that all of the object has been removed.

– If the object is not visible, do not poke around the auditory canal with tweezers, since this can cause even more damage.

– Ask the individual to lean his head toward the side affected, to encourage the object to fall out through the force of gravity. Do not hit or shake his head.

– If the object still does not come out, call the doctor.

• If it is an insect:

– Do not let the individual touch his ear, since the insect might sting.

– His head should be inclined away from the affected side in the hope that the insect goes out by itself.

– If you are quite sure it is an insect, a little olive oil or baby oil can be poured into the ear. While pouring, move the lobe back and up, if the individual is an adult, and back and down in the case of a child. In this way, the insect may come out floating in the oil. Only use this method if you are sure that an insect has got into the ear.

How to prevent injuries to the ears

Given that children are the main victims of this type of injury, it is necessary to teach them not to put objects in their ears:

• Teach the child not to insert pencils or Q-Tips.

• Accustom the child to using ear protection when doing sports that might cause injury.

• Teach the child not to poke inside his ears to get rid of wax.

The auditory canal and eardrum are very delicate and can be damaged or bleed easily if a child pokes in his ear with a Q-Tip. You should explain to him that if he pokes in his ears, this can even push the wax further inside.

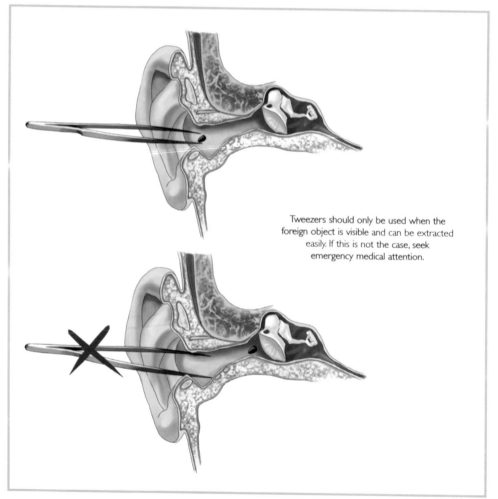

Tweezers should only be used when the foreign object is visible and can be extracted easily. If this is not the case, seek emergency medical attention.

Foreign bodies in the larynx and esophagus

The accidental ingestion of a foreign body is a potentially serious incident, which generally happens at home, and which on some occasions can even cause the death of a child. Avoiding this type of accident is much easier than dealing with its effects, which is why it is important to follow certain safety rules in order to avoid such mishaps, especially with smaller children.

What is a foreign body?

• A foreign body is some object, for example, a bone or the skin of dried fruit, that enters the organism via one of its orifices. This type of incident varies considerably in its degree of seriousness, since results can range from small local reactions to fatal accidents.

• The entry of foreign bodies into the organism is much more frequent in the mentally sick, nursing babies, people with neurological illnesses that cause problems in swallowing, and epileptics.

• Children less than three years old are usually the most common victims, although this type of accident can also occur in adults. Small children are at greater risk, since up to the age of three, they are very restless and want to touch everything

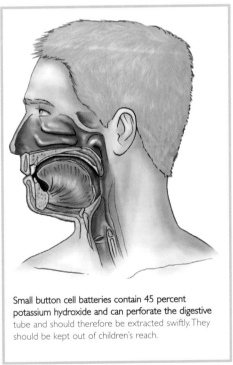

Small button cell batteries contain 45 percent potassium hydroxide and can perforate the digestive tube and should therefore be extracted swiftly. They should be kept out of children's reach.

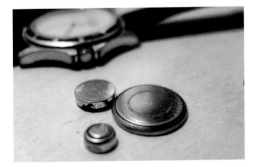

around them, and to use their sense of taste, they put many objects into their mouths. Furthermore, since their teeth are still undeveloped, they are unable to chew food properly and tend to swallow it whole.

Where might a foreign body become lodged?

When a foreign body has entered via the mouth, it may then go into:

- The respiratory ducts, passing through the larynx and trachea, even reaching the bronchial tubes.
- The digestive system, reaching the esophagus, the stomach, and both small and large intestines.

What are the most frequent objects that can enter the larynx and esophagus?

- The mouth and pharynx can easily be routes of entry for small, pointed foreign bodies such as, for example, splinters of bone, fish bones, toothbrush bristles, needles, pins, nails, coins, and fragments of wood and glass, which usually stick on the tonsils, at the base of the tongue, or sideways in the pharynx.

- Foreign bodies with sharp, pointed edges or those of large size can become blocked and lodged in the larynx.
- The trachea and bronchial tubes can trap dried fruit, needles, nails, buttons, coins, small rubber balls, food such as peas, fragments of plastic, etc. Normally, they lodge in the main right bronchial tube, since it creates a minor angle of deviation with the trachea.
- Finally, they can reach the digestive tract, given that children, if they are under three years old, often swallow coins, small toys, or pieces of toys.

What are the symptoms?

- In the mouth and pharynx, there is pain during swallowing, which can vary from moderate to intense, becoming extremely painful in some cases.
- In the larynx, it normally produces coughing, punctures in the throat and difficulty in swallowing. In some children, it can cause difficulty in breathing. If the foreign body is large in size, there is the danger of asphyxia.
- It also causes fits of coughing in the trachea and bronchial tubes as well, intermittent or permanent problems in breathing, pain, and a bluish

Adults are prone to swallowing bone fragments, glass, fish bones, fragments of dentures, needles, pins, nails, or stones of fruit.

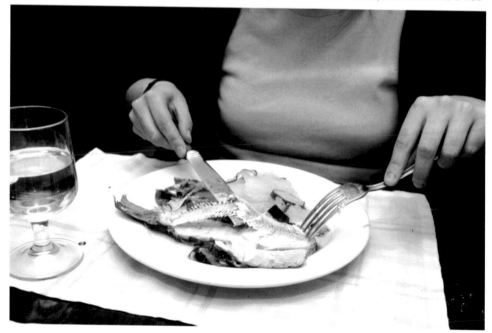

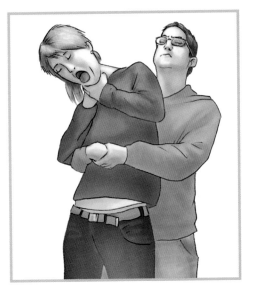

If a person suddenly shows signs of asphyxia and difficulty in breathing, you should immediately carry out the Heimlich maneuver.

skin color. If the foreign object has completely blocked the airways, it is a life-threatening situation.

What should be done?

• If a child puts something in her mouth, you must avoid shouting and remain calm. Shouting frequently scares children and they may swallow the object abruptly. It is also not advisable to put your fingers in their mouth. Generally, it is more useful to ask the child calmly to give the dangerous object back.

• If the foreign body lodges in the mouth and pharynx, it should be extracted as soon as possible; for this, you should seek medical help. If the object remains lodged for some time, there is a risk of injuries to the mucus membrane.

• If the object lodges in the larynx, you should go to the emergency room so that it can be extracted by specialists using an endoscope. If the foreign body is small in size, it is sometimes expelled through coughing.

If the extraneous object lodges in the trachea and bronchial tubes for long periods and the air-

ways become inflamed and/or the coughing is accompanied by blood, you must go to the emergency room to extract the object by means of endoscopy.

• If the child has swallowed the object and has no difficulty in breathing, it is very probable that it has passed the esophagus. If he is given some food and does not vomit, the object has probably reached the stomach and there is therefore no need to worry. It is only necessary to go to the pediatrician and tell him what has happened.

How can these accidents be prevented?

• Keep nursing babies and small children away from objects that they might put in their mouths. Make sure that there are no small articles within their reach, for example coins.

• Prevent them from running, crying, or laughing with food in their mouths.

• Prevent them from eating small food items, like peanuts or popcorn.

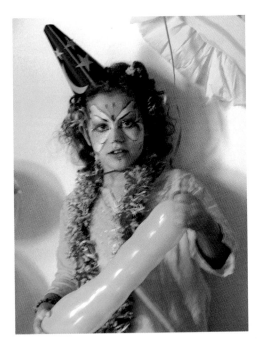

Small children should not play with balloons, since they are highly dangerous.

87

Burns

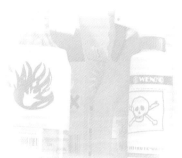

Most accidents to children happen at home, and among the most frequent are burns. These kinds of accidents, due to their gravity and consequences, require special preventive measures.

What are burns?

• A burn is defined as the loss of body tissue, caused by injuries to the skin and adjacent structures. When the burn is extremely serious, it can also damage the body's muscles and tendons.

• The majority of burns are caused by heat, in the form of fire or solar rays, liquids, or hot objects. Steam, cold, chemical substances, electricity, or radiation, are other possibilities.

• Burns caused by hot water, or liquids, represent one of the most common household accidents, especially with children.

• In the home, burns are a constant risk, since children can easily burn themselves with hot water,

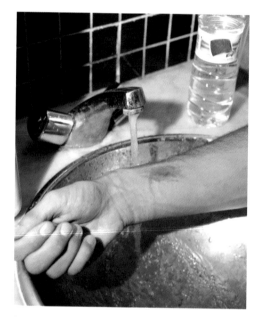

Superficial burns are painful, and the deeper they are, the less pain they cause, because the skin's nerves are destroyed. If the burn is red or blistered, or if it is superficial and painful, the prognosis is good.

The main symptoms of burns are the following:

• Appearance of blisters.

• Sensation of pain, which is not necessarily related to the seriousness of the burn: a serious burn might not cause pain.

• Peeling of the skin.

• Inflammation of the skin.

• In serious burns cases, the victim can become pale, their skin may turn cold and damp, their lips and nails bluish, and they may have a feeling of bewilderment.

• Also, in serious burns cases, the skin may appear charred.

or may suffer the consequences of an adult's actions (like spilling a cup of coffee or the contents of a saucepan).

• The seriousness of the burn and the effects of its general state depend on the temperature of the agent that caused it and the time that the victim remained in contact with the causal agent.

• The seriousness of the burn also depends on factors such as the location of the burn on the body, its spread and depth, as well as the age and state of health of the individual.

• Babies and children are more vulnerable to burns than adults, because they have a greater ten-

It is estimated that a high percentage of burns, around 85 percent, could be avoided, since they are generally due to domestic carelessness.

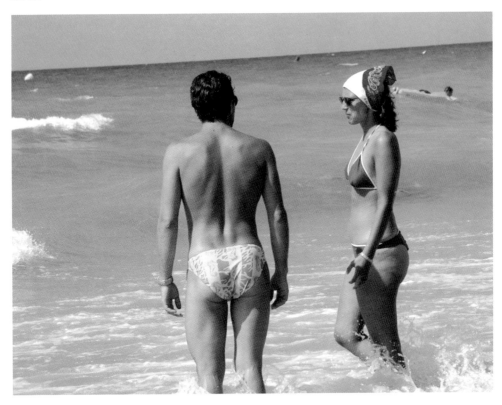

dency to touch household objects and their sensitive skin needs more protection.

• It is generally easy to avoid burns, by taking some very simple precautions to make the house a safer place.

• Burns can lead to minor medical problems, as well as life-threatening ones, depending on the spread and depth of the burn.

• First aid treatment varies according to the seriousness of the burn, its location, and the source of injury. Although minor burns are not a serious problem and can be treated without risk at home, more serious burns require medical attention.

What are the main causes and symptoms of burns?

In order to avoid possible burns, it is very impor-

tant to know their main causes, especially in children:

• The most common cause is contact with hot water, steam, spilt cups of coffee, and liquids that spill from pots, pans, and other kitchen utensils.

• Contact with hot surfaces or fire, for example, stoves, fireplaces, hair curling devices, etc.

The most common causes of first-degree burns are prolonged exposure to the sun or momentary contact with other heat sources.

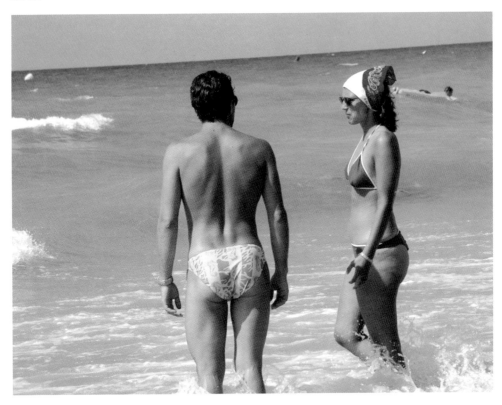

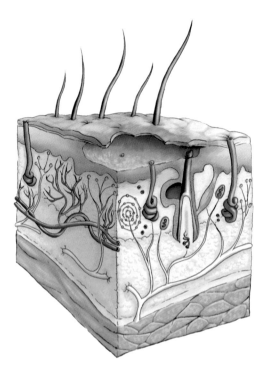

Cross-section of the skin layers affected by a first-degree burn. In this case, only the epidermis is affected.

• Batteries, whether alkaline or small button cell batteries, are among those chemical substances that cause burns. Cleaning products like those

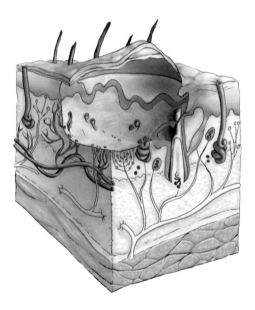

used to clean out pipes are highly contaminating, since they contain caustic soda, a very corrosive substance.

• Children have a tendency to bite electric cables, or put their fingers into sockets, which causes burning through exposure to electricity.

• Burns caused by excessive exposure to the sun.

Classification of burns and how to treat them

First-degree burns

First-degree burns affect the surface layer of the skin (epidermis); the skin reddens, becoming dry and painful, causing a burning sensation and becoming slightly inflamed.

If the burn has not affected large surfaces of the hands, skin, face, or groin, the following treatments can be carried out at home:

• Apply cold and damp compresses or towels, or submerge the part affected in clean cold water, though not excessively.

• It is also helpful to let the cold water faucet run over the burn. Continue until the pain passes, or at least for about 5 minutes.

• Try to calm a child who has been burned and tell him there is nothing to worry about.

• After the burn has been under running water, cover it with a sterile non-adhesive bandage, or with a towel, or piece of clean cloth.

• The burn must be protected from pressure or rubbing.

• Do not apply creams, since they may cause infection. When the skin has cooled, a small quantity of hydrating lotion can be applied.

• You can use painkillers such as acetaminophen (Tylenol) or ibuprofen to help alleviate the pain and reduce inflammation.

• First-degree burns generally heal without any further treatment. However, in the case of a first-degree burn that covers a large area of the body, or if the victim is a child or an elderly person, you should seek urgent medical help.

• Check if the victim has had a tetanus vaccine.

Second-degree burns are characterized by swelling and very intense pain. In addition, structures related to the skin are lost, such as hair (hair follicles), glands producing sweat (sweat glands), glands producing sebum (sebaceous glands), etc.

Second-degree burns

Second-degree burns affect the epidermis and its lower layer, the dermis. The skin becomes red and painful, blisters appear, it suppurates liquid, and the skin begins to peel.

In the case of second-degree burns, you should do the following:

• Apply cold and damp compresses or towels, or submerge the part affected in clean cold water, although not excessively. It is also helpful to let the cold faucet run over the burn. Continue until the pain passes, or at least for 10 minutes.

• After the burn has been under running water for a reasonable time, cover it with a sterile non-adhesive bandage, or with a towel, or piece of clean cloth.

• Do not touch the blisters.

• Do not apply creams, since this may cause infection.

• If the child is afraid, make him lie down with his feet raised.

• If the area of the burn is more than 2 inches (5 cm), seek medical help.

Third-degree burns

• Third degree burns extend to deeper tissue, making the skin change color, varying between white, brown, yellow, and even black, and feeling is lost due to the destruction of nerve endings. The skin dries up and has a tanned look. You can also observe swelling in the tissue.

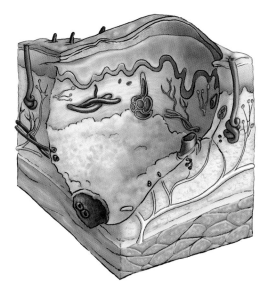

Without suitable medical attention, the healing process of extensive third-degree burns is slow and poor. Given that the epidermis and the hair follicles have been destroyed, the hair will not regenerate easily.

In the case of third-degree burns, follow this advice:

• Third-degree burns, if they are spread over a wide area, can endanger life. These injuries require immediate medical attention.

• In the emergeny room, staff will make sure that the individual can breathe well, they will check that other injuries are not life-threatening and begin treatment to replace lost fluids and avoid infection.

Chemical burns

• Burns caused by chemical substances can be very dangerous, because they penetrate the skin, damaging muscles, bones, nerves, tendons, and other important tissue.

• This type of burn constitutes one of the most complex emergencies to deal with, as much for the way different chemical products act, as for the great number of existing products in different spheres of life. It is estimated that currently there exist around 25,000 products for use in agriculture, industry or the home that are capable of causing burns.

• The majority of chemical burns occur accidentally, in most cases causing lesions of a minor nature that can be treated at home.

• Prevention is of vital importance with this type of burn. Employees should be made aware of the safety measures currently in force for dealing with hazardous products.

• Dealing with chemical burns, if these are serious, must be the function of specialized personnel.

What to do in the case of a chemical burn

• Verify that the cause of the burn has been eliminated. Place the burn under a faucet for at

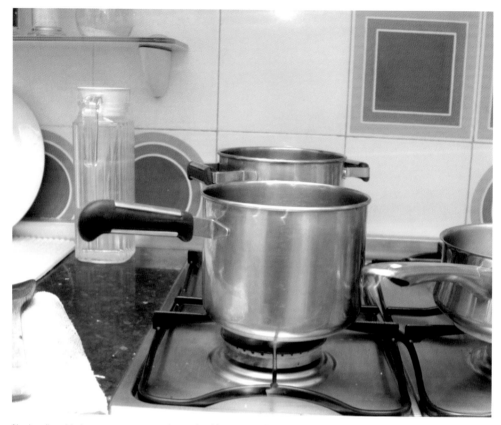

The handles of frying pans, saucepans, and pots should not protrude so that they can be knocked accidentally. They should always be kept pointing inwards.

least 20 minutes, to make sure that the chemical substance that caused the burn is washed away.

• Take off the clothing or accessories that are contaminated by the substance that caused the burn.

• Cover the burnt area with a dry sterile gauze or with a clean cloth.

• Wash the burnt area again for several minutes more if the accident victim says that the burning feeling has intensified after the first washing.

• Minor chemical burns normally heal up without additional treatment.

Normal domestic cleaning products, in particular those containing ammonia or bleaching agents, can cause serious damage to the eyes or skin, as can the chemical products used in gardening. It is advisable to read the product labels, which should contain instructions for their correct use and treatment recommendations in case of accidents.

When should medical attention be sought:

• If the chemical substance has burnt right through the external layer of the skin and the

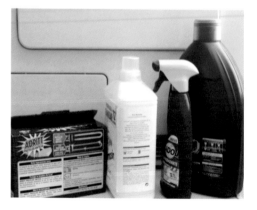

resulting burn covers an area greater than 2 to 3 inches (5 to 7.5 cm) in diameter.

• If the chemical burn has affected the victim's hands, feet, face, groin, buttocks, or a major joint.

In such cases:

• Take off all the victim's clothing and bathe him generously in water until the chemical substance has been completely eliminated.

• Do not stop pouring cold fresh water over the burn.

• Take the victim immediately to the nearest hospital, or call an ambulance to take him there.

Advice for preventing burns

• Whenever possible, place protection around hot objects.

• Use utensils that have insulated handles which are in good condition.

• Use insulating gloves or mittens to move hot objects or to handle them in a hot oven.

• Avoid splashes, using covers or lids while cooking food.

• Use stoves or burners set well back, away from the people using them.

• Do not serve food that is too hot.

• Do not hold children in your arms while handling hot liquids in the kitchen.

• Keep children away from the kitchen and the broiling area.

• Make sure hot objects or live flames are out of children's reach.

• Prevent children from playing with matches or lighters.

• Handle rockets, fireworks, and cartridges with great care and keep them out of children's reach.

• Do not place water containers on heating stoves or heaters.

• Keep the portable grill in a closed cupboard with the cable rolled up.

• Make sure sockets are blocked off by furniture.

• Keep electrical cables and equipment in good condition.

• Avoid the use of extension cables and do not overload sockets.

• Hide cables in corners or under furniture.

Allergies

Allergies are disproportionate reactions of the body to allergens. Allergies can cause illnesses, such as allergic rhinitis or asthma. Allergic attacks in the home can be reduced by following certain guidelines.

What is an allergen?

It is a substance that sensitizes the body and is capable of triggering an allergic reaction.

What are the main symptoms of allergies?

These symptoms vary according to the type of allergen and the sensitivity of the individual.

The following table shows the most common allergies:

What are the available treatments for allergies?

If you suspect you may suffer from allergy, you can consult an allergy specialist, who will perform the relevant tests to identify the allergens causing your symptoms and will prescribe the available treatment:

Antihistamine. Antihistamine reduces the main symptoms—sneezing, conjunctivitis. It is effective for all types of allergies. Second generation antihistamines do not produce undesirable

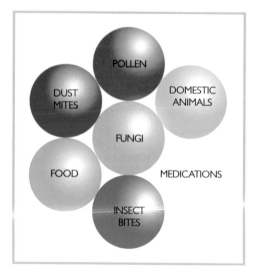

POLLEN

DUST MITES

DOMESTIC ANIMALS

FUNGI

FOOD

MEDICATIONS

INSECT BITES

Illness	Organs affected	Symptoms
Allergic conjunctivitis	Eyes	Tears, itchiness
Rhinitis	Nose	Nasal secretion, itching, sneezing, nasal congestion
Urticaria/Dermatitis	Skin	Stinging, reddening, edema, erythema
Bronchial asthma	Bronchial tubes	Coughing, wheezing, breathlessness
Anaphylaxis	The whole body	Itching, difficulty in breathing, reddening, sickness

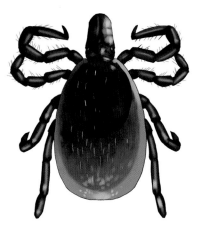

Mites are microscopic arachnids that live in the home and cause respiratory symptoms in individuals who are allergic to them.

What is histamine?

A substance released during an allergic reaction and responsible for many symptoms, such as a runny nose, conjunctivitis, and sneezing.

Corticoids. These are the most effective drugs for the treatment of allergic rhinitis, due to their anti-inflammatory effect. Corticoids in the form of nasal sprays are indicated for reducing the symptoms of rhinitis (running nose, itchiness, sneezing). They must be used regularly to be effective, even when the symptoms have ceased. They should not be used with children, or continuously for more than three months.

Cromoglycate. The use of cromoglycate is preventive and begins one month before the start of the allergy season. It acts upon the release of histamine.

Immunotherapy. In some cases, immunotherapy is carried out in the form of vaccines. This is used with patients who have very severe allergies that do not respond to medication. Small quantities of allergens are injected to make the patient develop immunity. It generally takes several months and has side effects.

side effects (first generation antihistamines tend to cause drowsiness, among other symptoms). They come in the form of capsules, creams, nasal sprays and eye drops.

Washing bed clothing with hot water once a week, and vacuum cleaning under the bed to take away the dust is very effective against allergy to mites.

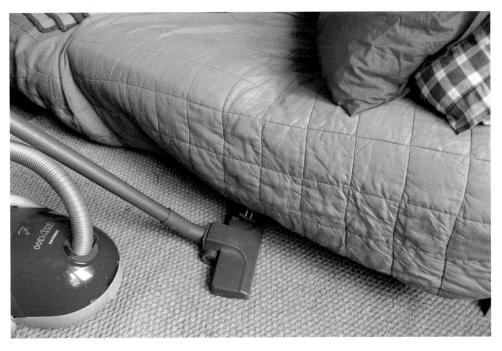

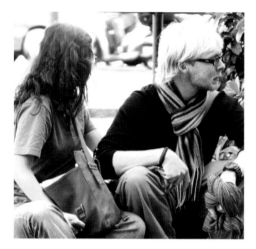

The symptoms of rhinitis caused by allergens are very similar to the common cold.

Allergy to mites

The majority of respiratory allergies (asthma and rhinitis) are caused by dust mites. The mites develop in warm and humid environments and feed on small microscopic fragments. They breed inside mattresses and pillows. Mites cannot tolerate low temperatures and do not exist at high altitudes.

Advice to follow at home for someone allergic to mites

• Use a vacuum cleaner with an anti-mite filter.
• Use an air-conditioning system of a closed air type, or with a changeable air filter. Change the filter at least four times a year.
• When cleaning away dust, use a damp cloth and a mask to protect your nose and mouth.
• Remove the carpets and rugs from the allergic person's room.
• Remove large curtains and other objects that accumulate dust.
• Do not decorate the house with textile objects.
• Use latex or foam mattresses or cover them with a special undersheet for allergy sufferers.
• Keep the house clean.

When you are outside, you accumulate allergens on your clothes and hair. If you want to get rid of them completely, when you get home you need to take a shower and wash the clothes you have been wearing.

Allergy to pollen (hay fever)

Allergy to pollen, also known as hay fever, appears with the following symptoms:

• Sneezing, nasal secretions, itchiness, nasal congestion (rhinitis).
• Tears and itchy eyes (conjunctivitis). It is easy to get confused between common cold symptoms and those of allergic rhinitis.

Advice to follow at home when living with a hay fever sufferer:

• Use air-conditioning systems with an anti-pollen filter.
• Keep the windows closed during the hours that have the highest pollen count (at dawn and dusk).
• Change your clothes and shower when you get home.
• Take the carpets and rugs out of the allergy sufferer's room.
• Remove large curtains and other objects that accumulate dust.
• Use a latex or foam mattress, or cover it with a special undersheet for allergy sufferers.
• Keep the house clean.
• On car journeys, close the windows.

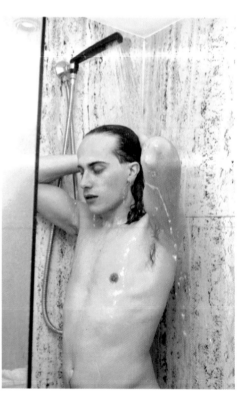

Advice for living with someone who is allergic to a certain animal at home:

- Keep the animal outside the house.

- If that is not possible, keep it away from the allergy sufferer's room and from the living room.

- Remove the carpets and rugs from the sufferer's room.

- Remove large curtains and other objects that accumulate the animal's hair.

- Use a latex or foam mattress or cover it with a special undersheet for allergy sufferers.

- Clean the animal's fur often and clean the places it normally goes.

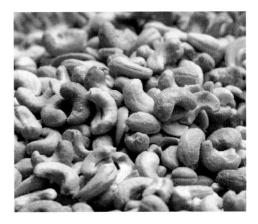

Peanut allergy is one of the most common food allergies, followed by gluten allergy.

Allergy to animals

The hair and skin of animals contain allergens that can produce very serious symptoms in certain people. The animals most likely to cause allergies are cats, but other animals, such as dogs, horses, and rabbits, can also cause allergies.

In the case of allergy to a certain animal, you must keep the areas frequented by the allergy sufferer clean and also the normal resting places of the animal.

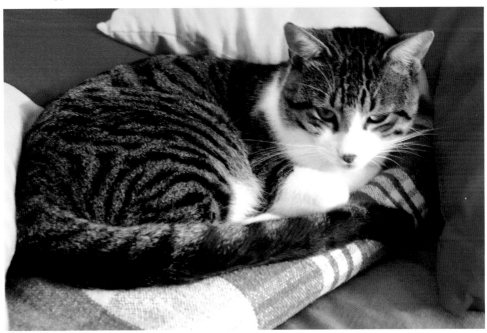

Advice for food allergy sufferers:

- Avoid the food in question.

- Ask about the ingredients of the food you eat. Sometimes, a certain allergen can be concealed in prepared food. Food allergy sufferers should ask about ingredients when eating out, or in restaurants.

- Read food labels.

- Be prepared for emergencies. Anaphylactic reactions to food can be life-threatening which is why people with serious allergies should take their medication with them to treat any reaction due to accidental ingestion.

- Wear a bracelet with details of your allergy.

In general, the symptoms caused by animals are:

- Respiratory symptoms (rhinitis, runny nose, sneezing, asthma, etc.).
- Cutaneous symptoms (skin inflammations).

Food allergies

According to statistics, 15 percent of the population are allergic to certain foods. The usual symptoms of allergic reaction to foods are:

- Respiratory symptoms; asthma.
- Swelling in the mouth.
- Digestive symptoms: diarrhea and vomiting.

The foods most commonly causing allergic reactions are:

- Cow's milk.
- Eggs.
- Fish and shellfish (prawns and oysters).
- Dried fruit.

Allergy to drugs

Some people can suffer allergic reactions caused by certain medications. Allergies to a particular type of medication are not usually different from food allergies or those related to other substances.

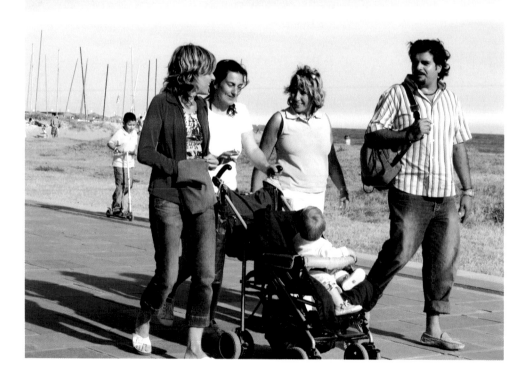

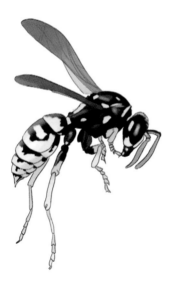

So far we have no evidence that wasps transmit disease, but if they sting someone who is allergic to them, the consequences can be fatal.

Advice to people who find they are allergic to a medication

• Do not take the drug that caused the allergic reaction again under any circumstances.

• If it was a prescribed drug, tell the doctor who prescribed it and see if there is an alternative.

• Keep the package containing the medication—it may be useful if you need to see a doctor following your attack, or for future reference so that you can avoid a repeat occurrence.

Around five percent of the population suffer from this type of allergy. Antibiotics are the medications that cause most allergic reactions, among them:

• Antibiotics (especially penicillin).
• Some types of analgesics.
• Local or general anesthetics
• Muscular relaxants.

Can you be allergic to an injected medication and not be allergic to the same medication taken orally?

When you are allergic to a certain drug, it should not be administered in any way, not even topically (creams, drops, etc.) because the reaction will be the same.

When cooking in the open air, keep all containers closed to avoid insects approaching and possible stings.

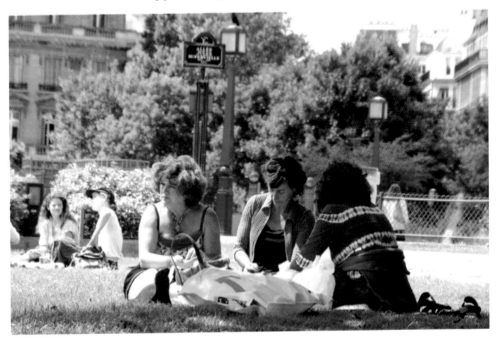

How to avoid insect bites

- Avoid going to the countryside in spring or summer.
- Do not walk barefoot in the countryside.
- Do not wear clothing with bright colors or flower patterns in the countryside.
- Keep trash bins tightly closed.
- Do not frighten insects away when they approach.
- Keep away from bees' and wasps' nests.

	COLD	ALLERGIC RHINITIS
Cause	Virus	Allergens
Appearance	Slow	Rapid
Duration	7–10 days	Brief (min/hours)
Frequency	Occasional	Recurrent
Nasal secretion	Dense	Watery
Pain in the throat	Frequent	Rare
Body temperature	Raised	Normal
Eye symptoms	Rare	Frequent
Coughing	Frequent	Rare
Sneezing	Frequent (but isolated)	Multiple (with frequency)

Allergy to insect bites

It is very common to get an insect bite, especially from a bee or wasp. Most people suffer minor pain and discomfort that only lasts a few hours at most. The affected area can become red with stinging and inflammation. However, there are some people who are allergic to insect bites because their immune system reacts disproportionately to the poison injected by the insect. It is not a very common allergy, affecting around one percent of the population.

Symptoms and what to do in the case of an allergic reaction

When a person is allergic to insect bites, the symptoms are usually very serious, since these bites can be a matter of life or death. Furthermore, the symptoms can spread in a few seconds to all the organs. This reaction is called anaphylaxis. The symptoms of anaphylaxis are the following:

- Extended urticaria (itching, burning, stinging) over the whole body.
- Inflammation of the throat and tongue.
- Difficulty in breathing.
- Nausea and vomiting.
- Diarrhea.
- Abdominal pain.
- Fall in blood pressure with shock and loss of consciousness.

If these symptoms occur, the patient should be taken immediately to the emergency room

Falls

People injure themselves easily. It is not a matter of age: children, adolescents, or adults may all have an accident that causes trauma. Among the most common form of accident traumas are bruising, sprains, fractures, and dislocations. This damage to the muscular-skeletal structure is very debilitating and painful. The degree of danger depends on the extent of the injury and the appropriate specialized treatment.

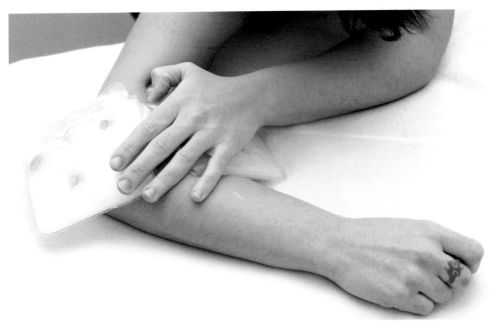

Applying ice packs on the injured area causes narrowing of the blood vessels, and anesthetizes the nerve endings.

Bruising

What is bruising?

Bruising occurs after being hit by a blunt object. This type of injury only affects the soft tissue, that is to say the skin and muscles. Normally, when you are hit by something, the blood vessels of the muscles are crushed superficially in the area closest to the skin. The severity of a bruise depends on where the blow has been received.

Bruises can be divided into two types:

- **Minor bruising.**

The injury is superficial, only causing the rupture of small blood vessels, appearing in the form of hematomas (collections of blood under the skin), making the area red.

- **Serious bruising.**

The injury is bigger and causes the rupture of larger blood vessels. Muscle, nerves, or bones may be affected by the injury.

	Minor bruising	Serious bruising
Pain intensity	Pain intensity is variable; depending on the area of the body where the blow landed	Very intense pain increasing when the affected area is moved
Inflammation	Variable inflammation	Inflammation visible to the eye

What are the symptoms of bruising?

The symptoms of bruising can easily be recognized:

- The injured area becomes inflamed and swells.
- Hematomas appear, although their presence depends on the depth of the blood vessels.
- Pain in the affected area.
- The presence of a lesion or damage to the skin.
- Sensation of tension in the muscle and skin.

What should be done in the case of bruising?

- First, reduce the pain. To this end, put an ice pack (never put ice on directly) on the affected area for about 15 minutes.
- Keep the injured area immobile.
- If there is a wound, wash it with running water; do not apply creams or ointments. Disinfect the wound with iodine or alcohol.
- If there is no wound, apply an anti-inflammatory and analgesic ointment.
- If the bruising is serious and has occurred in the leg, keep the leg raised for several hours.

- Do not massage the affected area vigorously or rub it.
- Do not drain the hematomas or squeeze them.
- For 48 hours following the bruising, you can alternate the application of cold and heat to the injured area.
- Acetaminophen (Tylenol) or ibuprofen may be taken for the pain. Aspirin is not recommended, since this can increase the size of the hematomas (bleeding under the skin).
- If the pain persists and you cannot move the injured area, go to a medical center.

How can you prevent bruising?

To prevent this type of injury is very difficult, since you cannot predict when you are going to receive a blow. However, it is possible to adapt your home to the needs of those who live in it; this is very important in the case of senior citizens.

- The home of an elderly person should meet a series of safety requirements:
- Make sure the floor is not slippery and fix the carpets down well in order to avoid tripping and falls.
- Use rubber-soled slippers that secure the feet well.
- Install a rail on the stairs.
- Keep the living areas in the home well illuminated.
- In the case of rooms with different levels, make sure steps are clearly indicated.

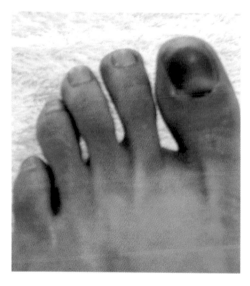

Hematomas are visible symptoms of bruising, but should not be confused with bruises, since hematomas can also be caused by different injuries, such as fractures or dislocations.

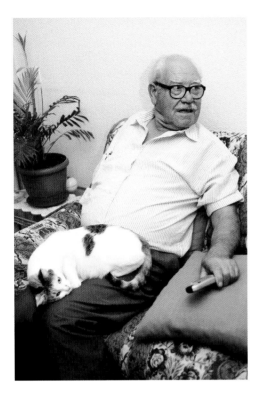

Home safety recommendations must be followed to avoid falls, since particularly for the elderly, they can have very severe consequences such as fractures, bruising, loss of mobility, loss of mental capacity, etc.

The most common dislocations occur in the shoulder, elbow, wrist, knee, and finger.

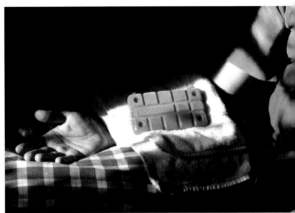

Ten percent of dislocations are combined with fractures with accompanying symptoms in addition to those of dislocation.

Dislocations

What are dislocations?

Dislocations are distensions of the ligaments and the socket where the bone lodges, causing the bone or the joint to become displaced. Any joint can become dislocated, although some are more susceptible than others, such as fingers, elbows, and shoulders.

What are the symptoms of dislocation?

• The first symptom is usually very intense pain, accompanied by swelling.

• Inability to move the joint or very reduced movement; in the most severe cases, the joint is visibly out of position.

• The pain is so intense that it is sometimes causes fainting. Later, the faintness tends to diminish.

• The swelling is so large in some cases that the dislocated limb looks deformed.

• Inflammation and reddening of the injured area.

Why do dislocations occur?

Dislocations usually occur as a result of abrupt movements, blows, muscular overload, and fatigue. The movement has to be in the opposite direction to the natural movement of the joint to cause dislocation. As a consequence, the ligament stretches so much that it reaches breaking point.

What should be done in the case of a dislocation?

In general, avoid touching the affected area and go to hospital for medical assistance. In the meantime, follow a series of additional steps:

• Apply ice wrapped in cloth to the affected area.

• If the bone has gone back into place, you can bandage it very gently without squeezing.

• Do not rub the affected area.

• Do not try to put the bone back into position.

• Take the person to a medical center, making sure they do not lean on the affected area.

SYMPTOMS OF SPRAINS				
	Pain	Swelling	Bruising	Joint movement
Grade I	Moderate	Moderate	Appears after the injury	Yes, with difficulty
Grade II	Intense	Severe	Appears immediately	Yes, with much difficulty
Grade III	Very intense	Very severe	Appears immediately	No

Sprains

What is a sprain?

When the joint ligaments break partially or totally, a sprain occurs. Sprains are responsible for 15 percent of all injuries associated with sports. The most common sprains are those of the ankle and wrist.

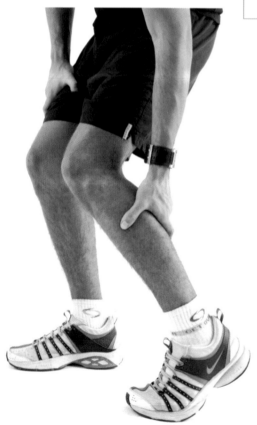

■ There are three types of sprains

- Grade I, or partial. The ligament is over-stretched and only a few fibers break.
- Grade II, or complete. The ligament breaks completely.
- Grade III, or dislocated joint. The broken ligament is accompanied by displacement of the bone.

What should be done in the case of a sprain?

- Apply an ice pack or cloth containing ice to the affected area; do not apply ice directly.
- Rest the limb affected.
- Take the casualty to the nearest emergency room.

Sprained ankles

Sprains are the most common injuries to the ankle. As with any kind of sprain, the ligaments become stretched or break partially or totally. The general advice above should be followed: cold applications, immobilizing the foot, and going to the emergency room. The time taken for recovery depends on the severity of the sprain.

Traditionally, with serious sprains, the foot was set in plaster and crutches were used for walking. Nowadays, the recommendation is for 24 hours' rest and a slow return to normal activity with the foot.

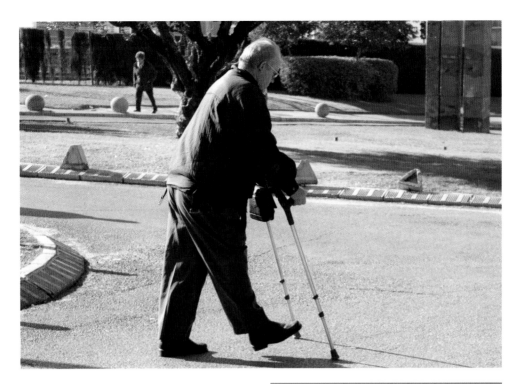

After a period of rest for 24 hours, you are advised to begin walking with a functional treatment bandage (or crutches, where necessary) and start progressive exercises to recover balance and mobility.

Fractures

What is a fracture?

Fractures are caused by an excessive and direct force upon the bone, causing it to break. Often, the fracture also causes injury to the soft tissue located around the fractured bone. In healthy people, fractures are generally caused by blows, although they can also be pathological: some people have an illness that causes bones to break without any blow being received. This can also happen in the very elderly, due to bone weakness typical of their age.

Fractures can be classified into two main types:

• **Simple fractures:** The bone breaks, but the skin is not affected.

• **Compound fractures:** The bone breaks, protrudes out of the skin, causing a wound. This can cause hemorrhage and infections.

What are the symptoms of fractures?

- Very intense pain. The pain is usually located in the area of the fracture and increases when you try to move the affected limb, or when pressure is exerted, however light.

- You are unable to move the affected area, due to the fracture itself and the pain it causes.

- A sensation of roughness, caused by friction between the fractured bones.

- Deformation and swelling of the affected limb.

- Hematoma (blood under the skin). This is caused by the rupture of the vessels located around the fractured bone.

- Fever. This can occur in young people and in the case of serious fractures, without any infection being present. It can also appear during the process of re-absorption of the hematoma.

What should you do in the case of a fracture?

Most fractures can be satisfactorily treated and recovery is complete. To achieve this, it is very important for the fracture to be immobilized and for a series of recommendations to be followed:

• Soothe the pain by applying ice packs or cloths containing ice to the affected area.

• Ensure that the casualty remains in the most comfortable position, avoiding any movement whatsoever.

• Do not try putting the broken bone back into position.

• Loosen the casualty's clothing, but do not remove it. This should be done by specialized personnel.

• Take the casualty to the nearest emergency room. If you think it is appropriate, call an ambulance, or transport the casualty yourself, supporting the injured part of his body upon a small board.

• If the fracture is compound, wash it with running water if possible, and cover the area with a sterile gauze.

• Do not poke around in the wound.

• Ask the casualty if he is vaccinated against tetanus.

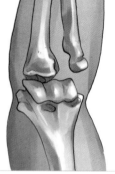
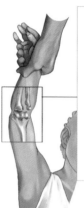

Experts are able to determine which bone is fractured, and where, by observing the deformation.

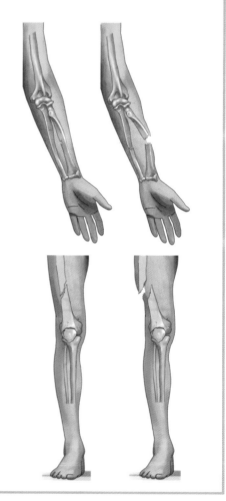

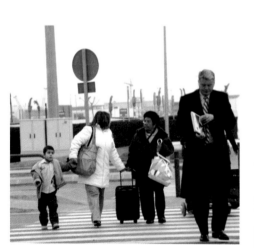

Electrical accidents

The increasing use of electrical devices in many activities and spheres of daily life—in industry, in the home, in transport, etc.—requires familiarity with certain practical guidelines. Electricity brings innumerable benefits, but it can also bring the risk of electrical accidents, not only to people, but to property and domestic animals. In order to prevent these accidents, it is necessary to adopt protective measures.

Injuries from electrical accidents

• When an electric current passes through the body, it causes electrical injuries, since the body closes the circuit by which the current enters and leaves.

• Exposure of the body to electricity causes three types of injury:

– Electrical burns. These are injuries caused by the thermal effect of the electricity. This type of injury is very dangerous, since the electricity passes through all the tissue of the body, the blood vessels, and nerves. The heat causes destruction of the tissue.

– The tetanizing effect. The electricity causes an over-stimulation of the cells, producing very violent muscular contractions, which can lead to fractures and dislocations in the joints and bones.

– Electrocution. The cellular over-stimulation also affects vital organs, such as the heart, lungs, or brain. An electrical accident can cause a cardiac and respiratory arrest.

If a fire caused by electricity occurs, do not use water to put it out; use an appropriate fire extinguisher.

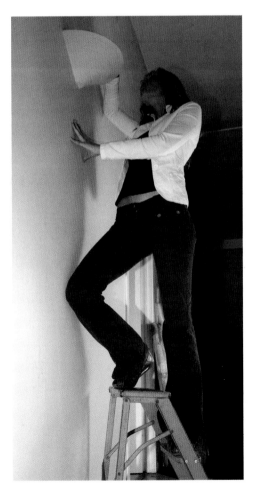

Electrical injuries can occur suddenly, for example in the form of electrocution.

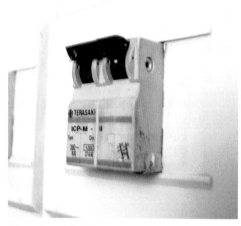

All members of the family should know how to shut off the electricity at home, and where this can be done.

The main causes of electrocution are people touching the exposed wires of electrical devices that have not been properly connected, or children putting scissors or wire into socket holes.

What to do in the case of an electrical accident

• Call the emergency services.

• Cut off the electricity before touching the casualty, either by disconnecting the supply at home, or calling your electricity company.

• If this is not possible, use insulated material, such as rubber gloves or wood to protect yourself from the electricity.

• Never touch the victim while he is in contact with the source of electricity.

• If the clothes of the casualty are burning, never extinguish this with water, use blankets and non-acrylic woolen clothing to put out the flames.

• Put sterile gauze over the burns. Before placing the gauze, wash your hands with soap and water. Do not touch the burn directly.

• If the casualty has stopped breathing, begin cardiopulmonary resuscitation procedures.

How to prevent electrocution in the bath

• Before handling any electrical equipment, your hands must be dry. This should apply at every

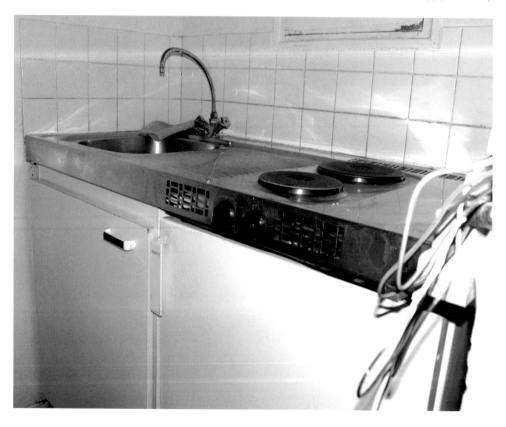

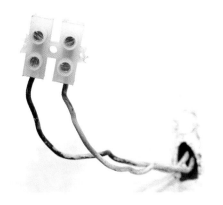

moment when you plug in, unplug, and turn on.
• Avoid walking barefoot or with wet feet when using electrical devices.
• Never touch electrical equipment when you are in the bath or shower.
• Make sure that an electrical device is quite dry before connecting it.
• Never disconnect electrical equipment by pulling the cable; this should be done by taking out the plug.

How to prevent electrocution in the kitchen
• Do not connect equipment that is wet.
• Read the manufacturer's instructions before using new electrical goods.
• Do not connect, touch, or use electrical equipment in your bare feet, even if the floor is dry.
• Disconnect an electrical device if you have to work on it.
• If any electrical device gives off a burning smell, or smoke, disconnect it immediately and call a technician to check it.

How to prevent electrical accidents when there are babies in the house
• Keep sockets out of children's reach.
• Do not touch sockets in the presence of children, since this can awaken their interest and curiosity.
• Do not buy electrical toys for babies. If a baby gets an electrical toy, watch him continuously while he is playing with it.
• Cover sockets with protectors or with insulating tape.

To change an electric bulb, first turn off the corresponding switch.

• Try not to let children play in front of the TV, because the cathode ray tube might explode if the television gets a knock.
• In children's rooms, do not leave cables or electrical equipment in a visible location.

How to prevent electrocution outside the home
• Avoid overhead electric cables, and prevent children playing with objects that can touch the cables, such as kites or model airplanes.
• When watering the garden, do not water near electric cables or meter covers.
• If any loose cable drops to the ground from a pole, call the electricity company.
• Do not enter huts where transformers are housed.
• Never go up high-tension pylons.

All the sockets in the house should be suitably protected, since they are the most common cause of electrocution in babies.

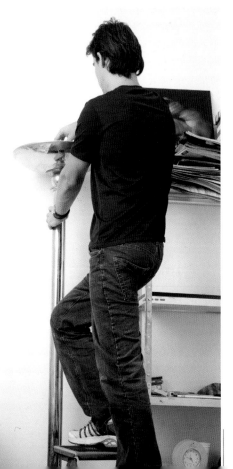

Bumps and bruises

Bumps and bruises are common occurances in the home. Children and the elderly are most prone to this type of household incident, so you must be extremely vigilant in protecting them.

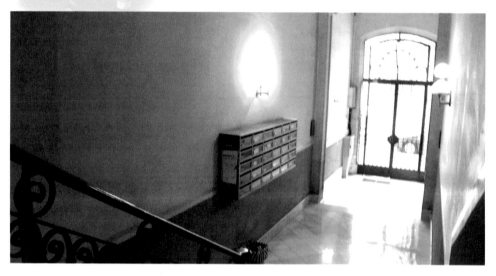

Bumps

How do we injure ourselves at home?
• At home, we can bump against fixed objects like furniture or the staircase, or moveable objects like doors and windows.
• We can also be hit by falling flowerpots, tool-boxes, or shelving.
• It is therefore important to control where these objects are placed, and also to monitor the areas we usually frequent and keep them free from obstacles (flowerpots, kitchen cupboards with open doors, etc.).
• This type of accident is very common and usually minor.

How to prevent getting bumps at home?
• Avoid leaving objects on the ground and keep things in order.

Broken teeth

This type of accident is very common during childhood. However, it is nearly always cause for a medical emergency. It frequently happens when a baby falls from his parents' bed or from the table where he is being changed, or when a child is older and practicing some kind of sport or playing around.

Suitable household lighting in areas people pass through, such as a corridor or entrance hall, helps to prevent unnecessary knocks.

Because children are so active physically, they get many knocks that can cause damage to their teeth.

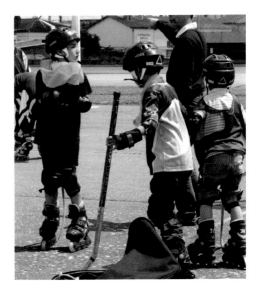

- Clean with anti-slip substances.
- Try to stop children playing on the stairs.
- Do not leave drawers or cupboards open.
- When acquiring decorative objects and domestic furniture, always choose those that have round edges.
- Place warning signs (stickers with a red circle, for example) on glass doors.
- Position hanging objects, like flowerpots, securely and at a safe height.

What should be done in the event of broken teeth?

- The speed with which a child's injured tooth is repaired depends on how quickly he gets treatment. If the whole tooth has come out, wash it with water, without brushing it, and place it in a glass of cold water or milk.
- Ideally, the tooth should not remain more than one hour outside the mouth, so that the damage can be repaired.
- If only a piece of tooth has come out, keep it as it may help in restoration.

- Check whether a piece of tooth is embedded in the lips, tongue, or cheeks.
- Wash the area generously with water.

Bruises

When a blood vessel bursts due to a bump, a bruise appears. When the blood vessel bursts, the blood spreads under the skin. The main symp-

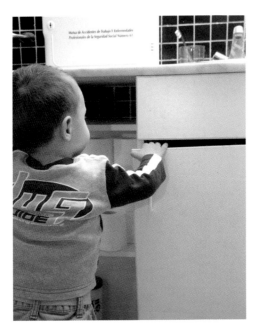

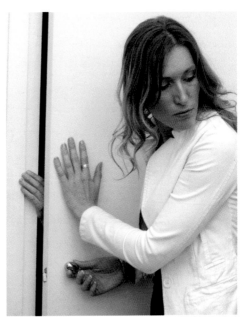

toms of bruises are pain in the area, inflammation, and change in skin color.

What should be done to alleviate bruises?

• Apply ice over the area to reduce the inflammation and speed up recovery of the bruise. The ice applied should be wrapped in a cotton cloth and have no direct contact with the skin. Keep the cloth ice pack on the skin for approximately a quarter-hour.

• To prevent the blood remaining trapped in the injured area, keep the area of the bruise above the level of the heart.

• Move the injured area as little as possible and do not put it under strain. In the case of children, do not allow them to run or do activities in which they use the affected part of the body.

• Do not touch the bruise or try to drain away the blood with needles or similar instruments.

When do you call the doctor in the case of bruising?

• If the bruise appears without any injury having occurred previously.

• If the bruise shows signs of infection (secretion of pus or fever).

• If it does not disappear within fifteen days.

Subungual Hematoma

Subungual hematomas (under the nails) are due to the accumulation of blood caused by the fingers

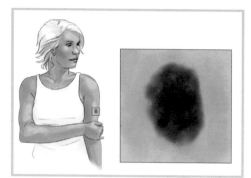

A hematoma is the accumulation of blood in tissue through rupture of a blood vessel.

getting hurt. The most common causes of this type of hematoma are trapping them doors. They are usually very painful.

◾ What should be done

Depending on the severity of the injury, it may be necessary to see a specialist. The hematoma may need to be drained and the finger should be examined to rule out possible bone injuries and carry out the appropriate treatment.

Development of hematomas

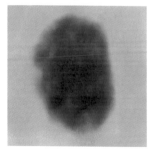

Hematomas usually begin as red or pink areas and are very sensitive to the touch.

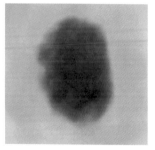

Later, they change to a dark blue or purple color.

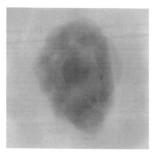

And finally, they turn green, dark yellow and light yellow, until they disappear. Hematomas normally disappear after about two weeks.

Wounds, cuts, and scratches

Wounds and cuts are injuries to the skin that cause pain, bleeding, and loss of sensitivity or function under the affected area. Wounds and cuts can be caused by sharp objects, such as knives, or by scratches producing a jagged look, or finally by pointed objects, such as nails. Caring for wounds aims to maintain hygiene in order to avoid infections that might worsen the condition.

What types of injuries are caused by tears and punctures?

• Tears have an irregular and jagged appearance. This type of wound occurs when the body's soft tissue is ruptured. They often become infected by bacteria and residue left by the object that caused the cut.

• Punctures occur through lesions caused by a pointed object, like a nail. Punctures also are prone to infection due to bacteria, but do not bleed as much as cuts. They also have a more closed appearance.

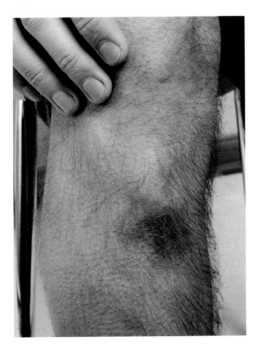

Differences between a cut and a puncture

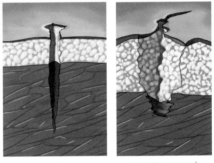

cut   puncture wound

What is a scab?

• When a wound bleeds, various specialized blood cells, called "platelets," come into action.

• The platelets coagulate around the wound, preventing further bleeding. The coagulation is formed by platelets and other blood cells that help to maintain its structure.

• Later, the coagulation begins to harden and dry up, forming a scab. Scabs are usually dark red or brown and look like bark.

• Under the scab, the damaged blood vessels repair themselves and white blood cells cleanse

The function of scabs is to protect the cut, keeping it free from bacteria and creating the ideal environment for the skin to regenerate under the wound.

113

What should be done with wounds?

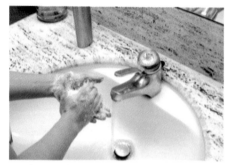

1. After washing your hands thoroughly with soap and water, to avoid infections, clean the wound, from the center to the outside, with soap and water.

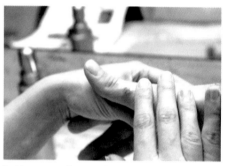

3. Use an antibacterial ointment to protect the wound from infection.

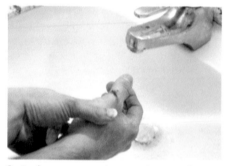

2. Apply pressure on the wound to stop the bleeding.

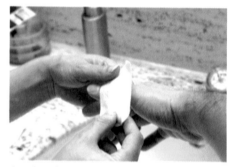

4. When the wound has stopped bleeding, cover it with bandages or dressings.

The stitches and staples should remain dry for a period, since the water might enter the incision and facilitate the growth of germs, thus causing an infection.

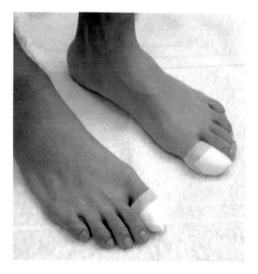

the dead cells around the cut and protect it from bacterial attack.

• As a result, a new layer of skin forms after one or two weeks. Until then, it is better not to touch the scab, since this can interrupt the healing process of the skin, damaging it again and delaying the process of scarring.

Wounds on the feet, punctures, and bites are those with the greatest chance of infection; they must therefore be treated carefully.

What is a scar?

• During the healing process of a wound, blood vessels form with the function of transporting additional blood to the scar, which causes its typical red appearance. On some occasions, the skin becomes raised and hardens. After about three months, the scar looses its red color and becomes flat. It will finally remain as a flat white line.

• If the wound has been large, the scar will not disappear, but it will become less visible than when the wound occurred. Some people's scars heal better than others.

• There is no method for accelerating the scarring process, although some specialists recommend the use of protective sun creams, since some scars redden under the sun's rays.

What is a keloid?

Keloids are tumors of the scar tissue. The body continues producing scar tissue for months or years, instead of the scar becoming flat and white over time. Keloids remain as red, hard, and raised scars. Surgery is necessary to remove keloids.

When should you call the doctor?

You should call the emergency services if the wound:

• is bleeding heavily, or the bleeding suddenly increases in volume, or has not stopped after pressure has been applied for 15 minutes .

• is very deep or very large, even if it is not bleeding heavily.

• is on the face or near to bones.

• measures more than about a quarter-inch (0.6 cm) and is big enough to be stitched.

• has been caused by an animal or another person, or rusty metal.

• has objects embedded in it.

• shows sign of infection (the area around the wound is red and painful, it is swollen, or has pus).

• Or if the injured individual has not received an anti-tetanus vaccination in the last ten years.

Caring for wounds after an operation

It is normal for a scar to become inflamed and red during the two weeks after a surgical operation,

If you follow the doctor's advice and maintain good hygiene, it is rare for postoperative scars to lead to complications.

although you should tell the doctor if there is suppuration, fever, intense pain, and/or abnormal sensitivity.

Strict hygiene is also very important when treating the wound:

• Wash your hands with soap and water after touching any dirty object. This is especially important after going to the toilet.

• The patient should ask people to wash their hands before touching him.

• If the patient is a smoker, it is advisable for him to quit smoking or cut down on cigarettes.

• The nicotine from tobacco slows down the healing process.

• The patient should not be visited by someone who is ill.

• If the bandage becomes loose, the doctor should be called so that he can put it back correctly.

What is tetanus?

• Tetanus is a disease affecting the central nervous system and is caused by the toxin of the bacteria Clostridium tetani. The spores of these bacteria are latent in the ground and are found all over the world.

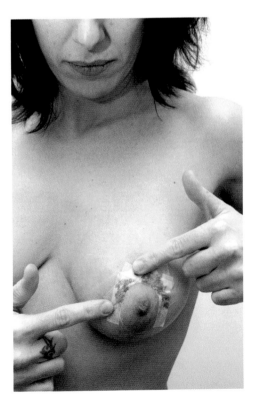

■ Caring for wounds after an operation

- Wounds produced by a surgical operation should be treated with the same attention as other wounds during the healing process, that is to say, with care—they should not be stretched or rubbed.

- Normally, on leaving the hospital, the incision is covered by a bandage. The bandages usually consist of gauze with plaster securing it.

- Generally, the incisions produced by operations should be kept dry for one week to ten days, until the stitches or staples are removed. If they get wet accidentally, they should be dried immediately.

- If the incision has been closed with suturing adhesive, it can be left uncovered and wet, although you must dry the area carefully after a bath.

- If the incision has been closed with suturing adhesive, it begins to lose adhesion after approximately two weeks. At this time and not before you can carefully remove any residue.

- If the incision has been closed with stitches or staples, the doctor is responsible for removing them after one week to ten days. This procedure is not painful.

- In case of doubt, consult the specialist, who will explain the specific care required for each type of incision.

- The disease begins when the spores enter the body through wounds or cuts. When the spores find a favorable environment in which to germinate, they begin to release bacteria that produce a toxin called tetanospasmin.
- Tetanospasmin causes spasms in the body muscles, which can lead to vertebral injuries, although it normally commences with light spasms in the muscles of the jaw, neck, and face.
- If untreated, the spasms spread to the muscles of the chest, abdomen, and finally the back. Sometimes the disease can affect the larynx, making even breathing difficult.
- One in three people if left untreated will die. This rate is higher in babies. The incubation period varies from 5 days to 15 weeks, the average being a week.

What are the symptoms of tetanus?

Tetanus causes one million deaths a year, especially in developing countries. The main symptoms are:

- Spasms and contractions of the jaw muscle. Later, spasms develop in other muscles such as the back, sometimes causing contraction of the chest, neck, abdomen, hands, or feet.
  - Convulsions.
  - Fever.
  - Sweating.
  - Irritability.

- Difficulty in swallowing, due to spasms in the larynx muscles.

There are four main clinical forms of tetanus, varying according to the severity, the origin, and the length of the illness.

- **Localized tetanus.** This is characterized by rigidity in the muscles around the infected wound. This phenomenon is attributed to the low toxicity

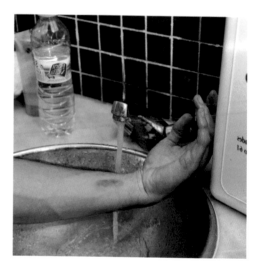

One of the most feared complications of any cut, bite, or other type of wound, however small, is infection by tetanus. Tetanus can develop over days or even weeks after the injury, giving rise to rigidity in the muscles of the jaw and other areas, and can even lead to convulsions and the inability to breathe.

What should not be done with wounds?

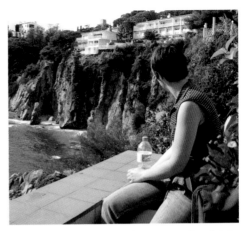

- Do not neglect hygiene. Although the injury might look clean and may not be deep, it should always be washed.

- Do not breathe or blow on an open wound.

- Do not remove embedded objects or sharp fragments from the wound; this procedure must be reserved for a medical specialist.

- Do not poke around in the wound or remove remains of tissue.

If you have suffered a wound, which has been exposed to the open air or been in contact with the ground and you have not received the tetanus vaccine for the last five years, go to a doctor immediately.

The tetanus vaccine, like all vaccines, can cause side effects, such as skin eruptions, inflammation, fever or headaches, but its advantages far outweigh these small inconveniences.

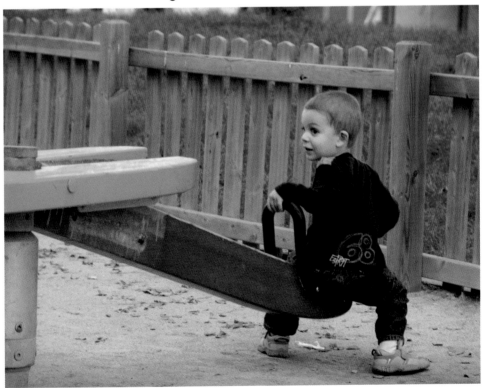

of the germ or to the partial vaccination of the infected person. The symptoms persist for weeks or months and disappear without any consequences.

• **Cephalic tetanus.** This rare form normally has a short incubation period (24 to 48 hours), the entry point being via the mouth and face and is characterized by paralysis of the muscles in the face or eyes and difficulty in swallowing.

• **Generalized tetanus.** This constitutes the most frequent and serious form of this disease, during which the classic symptoms of spasms and muscle rigidity appear. The principal muscles in the jaw are the first affected. The spasms or convulsions consist of violent muscular contractions that occur spontaneously or are triggered by different stimuli (light, cold, noise, touch, and food, etc.), possibly leading to asphyxia through lack of movement in the respiratory muscles. Recovery takes around 4 to 6 weeks, depending on the severity of the disease and the patient's response to treatment.

• **Neonatal tetanus.** This form affects new-born babies and the entry point is generally the navel where the umbilical cord has recently been severed. It has a short incubation period, the symptoms appearing possibly three days after exposure, at the latest on the sixth or seventh day. The first sign is difficulty or inability to nurse, developing rapidly into rigidity of the body followed by generalized spasms. The lower limbs remain extended and the upper ones bent

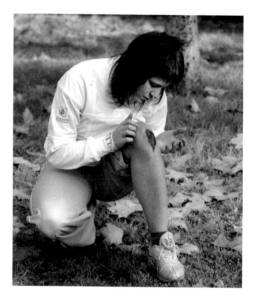

against the chest. The hands adopt a flexed position over the forearm with the fists firmly clenched, the eyes permanently closed in a wrinkled frown and the lips contracted.

Treatment for tetanus

The treatment for tetanus has several aspects: neutralization of the active toxin with a specific antitoxin, surgical cleansing of the wound, a peaceful environment that avoids even the slightest stimulus, tracheotomy (inserting a tube for breathing into the windpipe) when the convulsive episodes become a problem, and the administration of antibiotics.

▪▪ How to prevent tetanus

- Tetanus can be prevented by the tetanus vaccination. The vaccination does not protect against infection, but it protects against the effects produced by the toxin.

- The tetanus vaccination consists of three initial doses, a booster one year after the third dose, and periodical reminders to maintain protection.

- The general scheme is for five doses: at 2, 4, and 6 months old, at 15–18 months old, and then at 4–6 years old.

- In children under 7 years old (unless the anti-diphtheria or anti-pertussis (anti-whooping cough) vaccines are contraindicated) always receive combined DTaP (Diphtheria-Tetanus-Pertussis) vaccinations.

- For adolescents and adults, the single anti-tetanus vaccine (T) tends to be substituted by the Td vaccination, (anti-tetanus combined with anti-diphtheria), to maintain protection against both diseases at the same time. Children who have had DTaP will receive a booster of Td at about 12 years old.

Hemorrhages

The term hemorrhage refers to when blood escapes from inside the blood vessels (veins or arteries). Minor hemorrhages are a frequent occurrence throughout people's lives. Generally, this does not lead to any fatal consequences, although when a large amount of blood is lost, this is significant, putting an individual's life at risk or even causing death.

Blood vessels

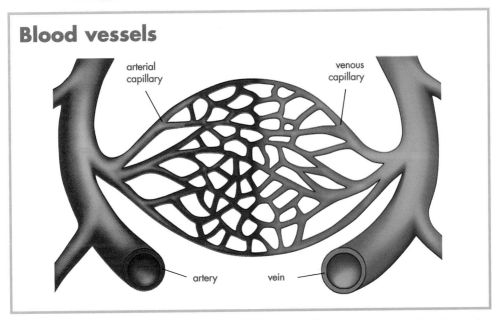

arterial capillary

venous capillary

artery   vein

The blood circulates inside the blood vessels (arteries, veins, and capillaries), which transport it throughout the whole body. When one of these vessels bursts, the blood flows out, thus causing a hemorrhage.

Hemorrhages

• When a hemorrhage occurs, all necessary steps should be taken to stop the loss of blood. If significant quantities of blood are lost, it can lead to loss of consciousness and may even end in death.

• Most injuries do not represent a risk to life, although certain rules should be followed to avoid later infections and other complications.

• There are three types of bleeding:

– **Capillary bleeding.** The capillaries are the smallest and most numerous blood vessels in the body. If, for example, a cut has occurred that severs a capillary, minor bleeding occurs. The blood's coagulation mechanism comes into action and the hemorrhage stops rapidly.

– **Venous bleeding.** Venous bleeding is blood on its way back to the heart, having already released its oxygen to the cells, which is why it is dark red in color. In this type of hemorrhage, the blood flows slowly and can be staunched by means of pressure upon the area.

– **Arterial bleeding.** Arterial blood is infused with oxygen and is bright red in color. In this type

To avoid serious wounds at home, you should keep knives and sharp objects out of children's reach.

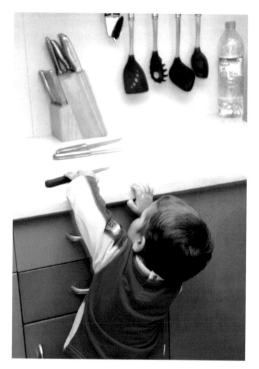

of hemorrhage, the blood comes out in rhythmic spurts, which coincide with the beats of the heart. This loss of blood is very dangerous. If the hemorrhage affects an important artery, it can lead to death in a few minutes. Direct pressure is also effective in this case, although recovery is slower than with a venous hemorrhage.

• Bleeding wounds can also be classified according to where they have occurred:

– **Internal hemorrhage.** This is when blood accumulates in an internal cavity of the body without reaching the outside.

– **External hemorrhage.** This is when blood leaves via the exterior of the body, whether from a natural orifice or from a wound.

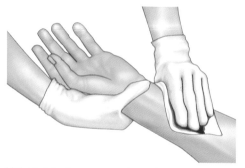

Method of direct pressure on a hemorrhage.

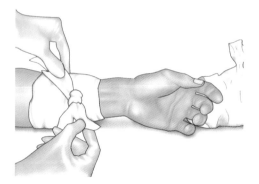

Other considerations regarding hemorrhages

• The severity of a hemorrhage depends on the speed with which blood is lost, the volume of blood lost, and the age and state of health of the person concerned.

• Among the causes of hemorrhages are cuts, punctures, grazes, violent tearing of the skin, etc.

• Serious wounds do not always bleed profusely, while other minor wounds, like those occurring on the scalp, bleed a lot.

• Puncture wounds do not bleed a lot, although they are dangerous due to having a high risk of infection: they therefore require medical attention.

• There are particular problems for hemophiliacs and people on certain medications that thin the blood. When such people hemorrhage, they tend

When the bleeding stops, bind the wound with a tight bandage and apply an ice pack for 10 minutes.

Pressure points between the wound and heart to stop hemorrhaging

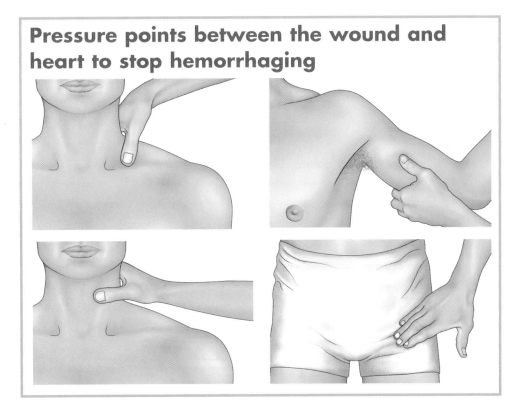

to bleed excessively. In cases like this, you should go to the emergency room immediately.

• Before treating a hemorrhage, wash your hands with soap and water and put on latex gloves. All first aid kits should contain latex gloves. Their use is very important to avoid the risk of contracting hepatitis or the HIV virus.

• It is imperative to call the emergency medical services if the hemorrhage is severe, if a part of the body has been separated, or the bleeding is accompanied by a head injury.

• The signs and symptoms of hemorrhages depend on the organ affected and the quantity of blood lost. However, the most characteristic symptom of all is the outflow of blood, both in external hemorrhages and in internal ones that manifest themselves externally.

• Hemorrhages are also often accompanied by other symptoms, such as paleness, cold sweats, accelerated heart rhythm, weak pulse, accelerated respiration, fall in body temperature, and, if not treated in time, loss of consciousness. If unchecked, death may occur.

What should be done in the case of external hemorrhages?

• Make the individual who has suffered the hemorrhage stretch out. If possible, the person's head should be lower than their trunk or legs, to help the flow of blood reach the brain. In this way, the risk of fainting is reduced.

• If the wound is on a body extremity, it is helpful, whenever possible, to raise the bleeding area in order to reduce the flow of blood. Elevating the injured part reduces blood pressure in the area of the wound and reduces bleeding.

• Local pressure should be exerted at the point of bleeding, with one or two fingers, or with the palm of the hand, using a piece of sterilized dressing suited to the size of the wound.

• If the bleeding does not stop, pressure must be exerted on the following arteries:

– Neck: carotid.

– Shoulder: retroclavicular.

– Arm: humeral (inside of the arm).

– Thigh: femoral (groin).

– Leg: popliteal area.

Tourniquets

A tourniquet is a procedure undertaken to control severe hemorrhagingthat cannot be contained by conventional means, using compression of the blood vessels in the immediate surrounding area.

Tourniquets should only be used in the following situations:

- When more than one accident victim has to be attended to.
- When a body limb has been severed or crushed.

Tourniquets are placed above the elbow or above the knee between the heart and the wound.

Once one has been applied, it should never be loosened.

After this has been done, it should be left visible, with a label indicating the victim's name and the exact time the tourniquet procedure was performed.

It is important to remember that tourniquets involve risks: gangrene may result, or even death from poisonous substances occurring in the body.

When the bleeding stops, ice should be applied (never directly) on the affected area.

If the bleeding continues or recommences after following all the above steps, go to the emergency room immediately.

▪ What to do

- The moment an internal hemorrhage occurs, the victim should go immediately to the emergency room, where they will try to control the hemorrhage and locate its origin, so as to perform the correct treatment.
- Avoid loss of heat in the victim, by covering him with a blanket.
- Do not give the patient anything to drink.
- It is possible that immediate medical intervention may be necessary to stop the hemorrhage, with medications, intravenous liquids, and even endoscopy or surgery.

Internal hemorrhages

Internal hemorrhage means that the blood does not flow to the exterior of the body, but remains in the interior, generally accumulating under the skin or in an organ cavity; this is the most serious form of hemorrhage.

- Causes of internal hemorrhage:
- Cancer.
- Cirrhosis.
  Polyps in the colon.
- Gastric complications.
- Hemophilia (defective blood coagulation).
- Leukemia (cancer of the blood).
- Aneurisms and other vascular disorders.
- Injuries.
- Signs indicating that an individual is suffering an internal hemorrhage:
- On palpitating the abdomen, it proves to be very sensitive or stiff.
- Hematomas are evident in different parts of the body.
- The person is losing blood via the rectum or vagina.
- The casualty is vomiting blood.
- Simple bone fractures (with no rupture of the skin) are evident.

Nasal hemorrhages

Nasal bleeding, also called epistaxis, is very frequent and the most common causes are bumps

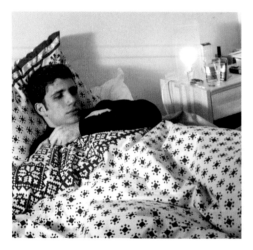

Most internal hemorrhages cause a constant loss of small quantities of blood. If undetected and left untreated, a concealed hemorrhage can lead to severe anemia.

to the nose, inflammation of the nasal mucus membranes due to allergies or other factors, wear in the mucus membranes, or breathing excessively dry air. Many cases of nasal bleeding occur without any apparent reason.

Most nasal hemorrhages originate in the nasal wall and are generally easy to stop. In some individuals, the nasal bleeding originates in deeper areas of the nose and this bleeding, which is less frequent, is very difficult to arrest.

Nasal hemorrhages can be an alarming occurrence, but they are not normally dangerous.

They are quite common in children, especially in dry climates or during the winter months; this is when the dry heat from household heating can cause dryness, cracking of the tissue or scabs inside the nose.

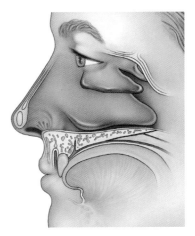

What should be done in the case of a nasal hemorrhage?

• If it is a child who is suffering the hemorrhage, you must reassure him and explain that help is at hand.

• Make the child sit down in a straight posture and lean forward, to prevent him swallowing blood. His head should be leant forwards, to avoid possible inhalation of blood clots. The sitting position reduces the blood supply to the head and nose.

• Next, in order to interrupt the hemorrhage, direct pressure should be applied upon the nasal orifice that is bleeding and against the nasal partition, pressure that is maintained for 5 minutes (timed). Do not slacken the pressure to see if the bleeding has stopped.

• Make the child breathe through his mouth.

• Do not expose the child to the sun during this period.

• After 5 minutes, release the pressure and check if the bleeding has stopped.

• Then, apply ice or a cold-water compress to

the bridge of the nose.

• If the hemorrhage has not stopped, repeat the earlier steps again.

• If the patient still continues bleeding after the earlier steps have been repeated twice, block the nasal passage by introducing a roll of sterile gauze soaked in oxygenated water, to act as a plug and stop the hemorrhage.

• Remove the plug after 4–6 hours.

• Do not allow the child to sleep.

• If the bleeding recurs, block the nose again with a plug and go to the doctor.

How to prevent nasal hemorrhages

Nosebleeds are normally isolated events; however, in certain children and adults they occur frequently. Certain household remedies can be used that may help to make hemorrhages a more rare occurrence:

• If the air in the house is not humid and the nasal passages become dry, a cold vapor humidifier should be used in the rooms where the air is driest, especially at night. Humidifiers collect germs and mold, and should therefore be cleaned thoroughly, according to the manufacturer's instructions.

• Apply Vaseline in the nostrils several times a day, especially at bedtime, to help keep the area moist.

• Use drops of saline solution (salted water) or a saline nasal spray, as indicated by the doctor.

• Teach the child not to poke up his nose, or blow energetically.

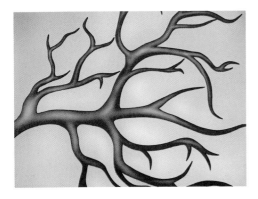

The frontal part of the nose contains many fragile blood vessels that can easily get damaged.
Most nasal hemorrhages in children occur in the frontal part of the nose around the nasal passages.

Steps to follow to stop nasal hemorrhages

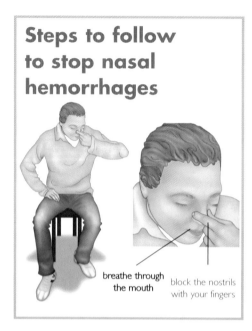

breathe through the mouth

block the nostrils with your fingers

Hemorrhages in the ears

Hemorrhages in the ears, also called "otorrhagia," consist of the outflow of blood from the ears.

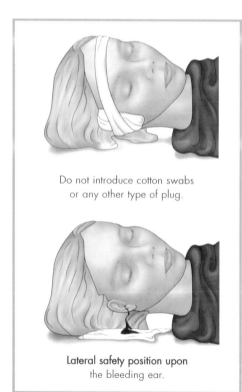

Do not introduce cotton swabs or any other type of plug.

Lateral safety position upon the bleeding ear.

These hemorrhages are rare and their origin is mainly trauma or severe inflammation.

What should be done in the case of a hemorrhage in the ears

• Make the victim lie down, so that the hemorrhage in the ear stops.

• Place a pillow under their head.

• Do not handle the ear or poke in it, since this can lead to infection.

• Take the victim to a doctor, ensuring that he remains in the recommended position.

Other hemorrhages

Gingivorrhagia. These are small hemorrhages in the gums that usually indicate a vitamin C deficiency disorder or an infection. They do not normally require urgent treatment.

Hemoptysis. These are hemorrhages originating in the lung. They are usually due to pulmonary diseases or chest injuries. They are recognized by the following symptoms:

• They appear with or after a cough.

• The blood is mixed with foam or bubbles.

• The color of the blood is bright red.

• The patient does not normally lose consciousness.

• Sometimes the patient notices a small tickle inside the chest.

What should be done in this situation:

• Absolute rest in bed in a half-sitting position.

• Do not give the patient anything via the mouth.

• Place an ice pack on the chest.

• Conserve the expelled matter for medical examination.

Hematemesis. This is a hemorrhage originating in the upper digestive system, principally the stomach. It can be recognized because:

• It is expelled externally together with vomiting.

• It is often mixed with food remains.

• The color of the blood is usually dark red, although not always; sometimes, it is expelled in the form of blood clots or particles resembling coffee grounds.

What should be done:

• The patient should rest in bed.

• Total abstinence should be adhered to, that is, no liquids or solids.

• Place an ice pack on the abdomen, above the navel.

• Conserve the vomit for examination by the doctor.

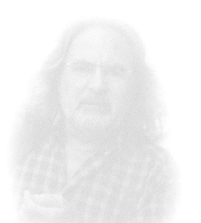

Poisoning

Poisoning is the result of the action of a toxic substance on the human body. According to the concentration, dosage, and the time of exposure to the substance, poisoning may be severe or chronic.

Poisoning via the digestive tract

The digestive tract includes the whole route along which the food we ingest is processed: the mouth, pharynx, esophagus, stomach, and finally the small and large intestines. Some of the principal poisons that enter the body through the digestive tract are:

- Contaminated water.
- Food in a bad state of preservation.
- Poisons (insecticides, rat poisons).
- Vegetal poisons (from mushrooms or herbs).
- Medications (overdoses, expired medicines).
- Cleaning products for domestic use.

Once the poison has been ingested, the victim goes through three symptomatic phases, depending on the location of the ingested poison inside the body:

– During the first phase, the poison is still in the digestive system, causing abdominal pain, nausea, vomiting, and diarrhea.

– During the second phase, the digestive system has already absorbed the poison and it has passed into the bloodstream, inducing fever, general discomfort, skin eruptions, and sweating.

– During the third phase, the poison has already reached the nervous system, causing alterations in consciousness, blurred vision, and convulsions.

What should be done in the case of poisoning via the digestive tract?

- It is very important to try to prevent the digestive system absorbing the poison, the best method being to induce vomiting. This should be done within the first three hours after ingestion of the poison.
- The most common method to induce vomiting consists of putting your fingers down your throat, as far as possible.

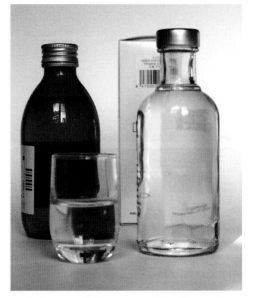

It is impossible to specify all existing poisons, since some substances, when used correctly, are harmless, but when used incorrectly, can become toxic (for example, alcohol).

- Another method to induce vomiting is to drink salty water in large quantities.
- Take the patient to the emergency room.
- DO NOT INDUCE VOMITING IN THE FOLLOWING CASES:
  – If there are burns on the lips and in the mouth.
  – If the victim's breath smells of kerosene, gasoline, or its derivatives.
  – If there are signs that the victim has ingested caustic products or turpentine.

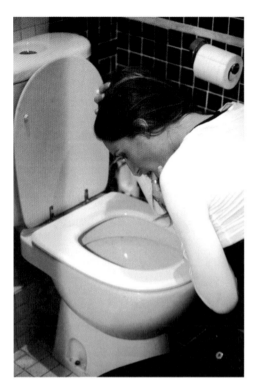

– If this is stated on the product label.
– If the victim is unconscious or has convulsions.
– If more than two hours have passed after ingestion of the poison.

What should be done in the case of ingesting caustic products

General rules:
• Never administer alkaline substances (such as sodium bicarbonate) in the case of acid poisoning, since the combination of both substances causes

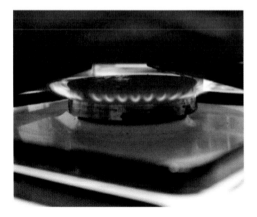

If you are sure that the individual has not swallowed bleach, caustic soda, or other caustic products, vomiting should be induced.

the formation of copious gases that lead to vomiting and can even cause a gastric rupture.
• In the case of alkaline poisoning, you should always dilute the poison by drinking liquids.
• You should only try to neutralize the substance with milk of magnesia in the first 10–15 minutes after the caustic product was swallowed.
• Take the victim immediately to hospital.
• Specific rules regarding the ingestion of acids:
• Do not make the patient vomit.
• Neutralize the acid with mild alkaline substances, such as milk or large amounts of water. In the case of powerful acids, these can be neutralized chemically by giving the victim a glass of milk of magnesia to drink.

Specific rules regarding the ingestion of alkalis:
• The alkaline substance most frequently ingested is bleach.
• Do not induce vomiting.
• Neutralize the alkali by getting the patient to drink dilute acetic acid, vinegar solution (1 part vinegar to 10 parts water), lemon juice, milk solution, or water with egg whites mixed into it (2 beaten egg whites in about a pint of water).

Caustic products

The word "caustic" comes from the Latin causticum, which means "burning."

It thus applies to highly dangerous substances, which destroy tissue upon contact and can cause death in a few hours or have significant consequences for the rest of your life.

They are a significant concern because the most frequently used caustic products are commonly found in the home and used for cleaning (detergents, deoxidants, bleaches, for example).

Kitchen stoves and gas heaters should be checked at intervals to avoid leaks that are dangerous to health.

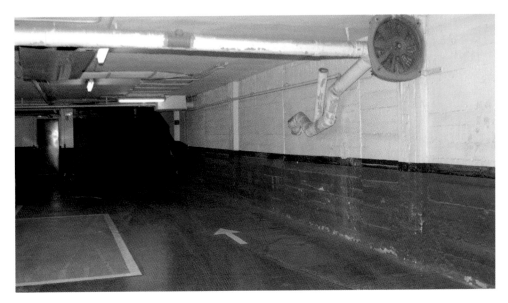

Garages in particular should be well aired or have ventilation systems that prevent the accumulation of gases.

What should you do if somebody has breathed in a poisonous substance?

• First, the victim should be taken away from the place where the poisoning occurred and, if possible, taken to a ventilated area.

• Before removing a person from a toxic environment make sure that you and whoever is helping are protected against the toxic atmosphere, whether with a mask, or with a damp towel placed over the mouth and nose.

• Take the patient immediately to the emergency room.

Inhalation of toxic gases

• The most common causes of inhalation of toxic gases are:

– Leaks of butane or other gas sold to the public, in the home, or in more ventilated places. Fortunately, these gases give off a characteristic odor, so they can be detected quickly.

– Stoves and heaters that malfunction can give off carbon monoxide, which is a very dangerous gas, since it does not give off an odor, or irritate the mucus membranes, thus making it very difficult to detect.

– Gases expelled by cars in enclosed spaces, for example, garages or other badly ventilated areas. This is potentially a very dangerous situation, since car exhaust pipes also discharge carbon monoxide, but fortunately exhaust pipes also emit odors coming from other kinds of gases and are thus more easily detectable.

Carbon monoxide poisoning

• Carbon monoxide is colorless, odorless, and tasteless.

• This gas is released through the incomplete combustion of malfunctioning stoves, through cigarette smoke, and from car exhaust pipes.

• Poisoning by this gas occurs in rooms without ventilation, tunnels, closed garages, and kitchens that have inadequate venilation for gas stoves.

• This poisoning is very dangerous, since it can cause death, particularly while sleeping in an unventilated room with malfunctioning gas appliances.

• When the victim is conscious, the symptoms caused by this poisoning are the following:

– Reduced reflexes.

– Intense headache.

– Vomiting.

• If the victim is unconscious, he will present the following symptoms:

– Flaccid and weak arms and legs.

– Difficulty in breathing.

– The skin turns pink.

– The eyes do not blink.

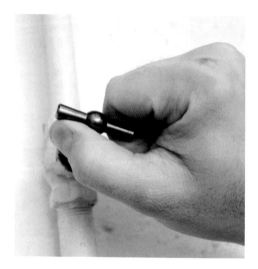

• If you suspect that the victim has carbon monoxide poisoning, he should be removed immediately from the room where he is and taken to a ventilated place.

• If breathing has stopped, cardiopulmonary resuscitation procedures should be carried out.

• Take the victim to the emergency room.

Poisoning by stimulant drugs, depressants, or those that affect the activity of the central nervous system

• These types of medications are of the sedative, anxiety-reducing, tranquilizing, or sleep-inducing variety.

• The symptoms will be different, depending on the effects and dosage of the ingested drug, although in general they are the following:

– The victim has difficulty in speaking and cannot be understood.

– His movements are uncoordinated—if you give him a glass of water, it will be hard for him to hold or he may drop it, he will not be able to walk in a straight line and will fall down easily.

– His breathing will slow down.

– His pupils will be smaller than normal and not react to light.

• In the case of this type of poisoning, you should:

– Talk to the individual to prevent him falling asleep.

– Move him to a safe place, to prevent him falling downstairs, cutting himself with knives, burning himself with lighted cigarettes, etc.

– Stay next to the victim and do not leave him alone at any moment.

– Take the victim to the emergency room.

Poisoning by anti-depressants, non-stimulants, or drugs that do not affect the central nervous system.

• The symptoms will be different, depending on the effects and dosage of the ingested drug:

– Given that the poisoning is via the mouth, nausea, vomiting, and diarrhea may possibly occur.

– Abdominal pain, headaches, vertigo, convulsions, and cardiorespiratory arrest (heart failure and breathing stopped).

• In the case of this type of poisoning, you should:

– Call the emergency medical services to collect the victim urgently.

– If the poison victim is conscious, try to make him vomit if less than one hour has passed since he ingested the drugs.

– Look for the container of the ingested drugs and take it to the emergency room for evaluation by medical staff.

Poisoning by medication

This type of poisoning can be accidental in origin, for example, when a child has gained access to the household first aid kit and has taken medication not prescribed for him, or deliberate, when adults have suicidal tendencies.

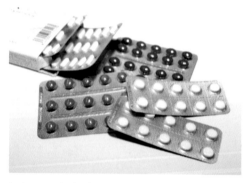

In the case of poisoning by medication, you should take the container of the drugs that were ingested to the emergency room.

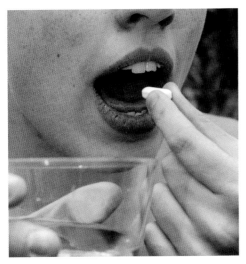

Acetaminophen poisoning can cause liver damage, which can lead to death.

— If the poison victim has vomited, collect a sample of vomit and take it to the emergency room.

Acetaminophen poisoning

• Acetaminophen, often known by the brand name Tylenol, is an analgesic and antithermal, that is to say, a drug used to reduce pain and fever. It is

Nearly all substances ingested in large quantities can be toxic. It is advisable to contact a toxicology center to get the latest information.

one of the most frequently used medications in children and adults and accounts for a considerable number of poisoning cases brought to the emergency room. Its toxicity is currently a significant cause of death in many countries.

• When administered in therapeutic doses as indicated by the doctor, it is generally well tolerated and safe, without producing any toxic effects. However, when you take five times the dose recommended by the doctor or more, a toxic reaction occurs that goes through different phases:

— It is important to be aware that the symptoms of this type of poisoning do not appear immediately, are very mild and give no warning of the severe symptoms occurring later, which are very serious and may cause death.

— In phase I, which takes place during the first 24 hours, nausea, vomiting, and drowsiness can occur, but some poison victims do not present these symptoms.

— In phase II, which occurs from between 24 and 72 hours, pain can begin to appear in the

Storing medications in high-up but visible places is counterproductive and can even cause children to fall when trying to reach them.

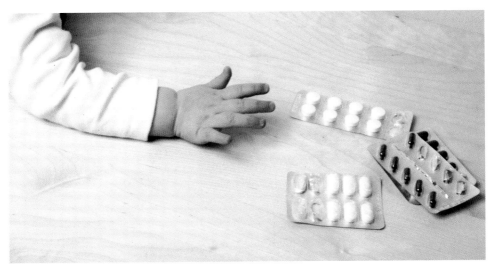

Preventive measures

- Do not store medications in places within children's reach.
- Do not mix medications with alcohol.
- Do not take medications from containers without labels or with illegible ones.
- Store such products in well-ventilated places.
- Do not mix cleaning products without first consulting the label, especially in the case of bleach and ammonia or hydrochloric acid, which give off the toxic gas chlorine.
  Label all cleaning products correctly.
- Do not spray insecticides and garden products on people, food, or domestic animals.
- Always use protective masks when working with aerosol paints and insecticides, etc.
- Wash your hands thoroughly with soap after using any chemical product.
- Do not remain in rooms that have been recently varnished or painted.
- Do not remain in rooms treated with insecticides.
- Do not keep your car running inside small, badly ventilated garages.
- Do not use stoves or burners in bedrooms.
- Turn off the gas supply after using it and also each night.
- If you smell gas, do not use electric switches, matches, or lighters.
- Do not consume food that has not been refrigerated properly.
- Do not consume canned food if it is bubbly, the can has perforations, or it has passed its expiry date .
- Throw away preserved food that when opened appears to contain strange substances.

right side of the body, where the liver is located. Some victims of this type of poisoning have difficulty in urinating.

— In phase III, which occurs from between 72 and 96 hours, the poison victim can present symptoms of jaundice, that is to say, their skin turns yellowish due to the liver damage caused by the drug. Between a quarter and half of victims have insufficient kidney function.

— In phase IV, which takes place between the fourth day and two weeks after ingestion of the acetaminophen, poison victims who have managed to survive begin to recover slowly. If treated in time, the liver lesions do not have long-term consequences.

How to prevent
acetaminophen poisoning?

- Unfortunately, the great majority of cases of acetaminophen poisoning happen in children who have swallowed it by accident. It is thus very important to keep this medication out of children's reach.
- Medications should be kept locked up.
- In the case of adults, they should remember that self-medication is a dangerous practice. It is always best to consult the doctor or pharmacist before taking any medication.

What should be done

The aim of the treatment is to reduce or limit the passage of the drug into the bloodstream once ingested, which can be achieved by inducing vomiting, preferably under medical supervision. In the hospital, the patient's stomach is pumped and a specific antidote is used, which, if administered in time, has the required effect. The most important thing is to go to the nearest hospital immediately.

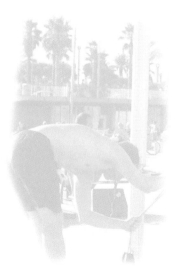

Muscular pains

Muscular pains usually come from overexertion or injury to a muscle after doing exercise or work that is not habitual. In these situations, the muscular pain tends to affect specific muscles or groups of muscles and its cause is fairly obvious. However, muscular pain can also be linked to other ailments.

What are muscles?

The human body has more than 600 muscles. Their functions are very diverse, from pumping blood through the whole body, to lifting objects or walking. Some of these muscles are controlled voluntarily, while others, like the heart, function in an autonomous manner. Each muscle is composed of thousands, or even tens of thousands, of little fibers.

• The heart is a muscle whose fibers belong to a special type, called "cardiac," because they are not found anywhere else in the body.

The muscular fibers of the heart are very resistant, contracting in a rhythmic way to pump blood to the whole body, and then relaxing again to receive more blood. The cardiac muscle functions like a smooth muscle, that is to say, in an involuntary manner. The heart has a group of cells, called "pacemaker cells," whose function is to control the beating of the heart.

• The skeletal muscles have the task of producing voluntary movements in the body, like for example, lifting weights. The arms will not move unless the body wants them to. Skeletal muscles are also known as "striated" muscles because,

▪ There are three types of muscles: smooth, striated, and cardiac.

• Smooth muscles move involuntarily: The brain and nervous system are responsible for sending the signals for them to contract.

• The stomach and intestine possess smooth muscles, which, with their contractions and distensions, help food advance through the body.

• Likewise, during the vomiting reflex, the smooth muscles of the digestive system come into operation, expelling food from the stomach, up through the esophagus and out of the mouth.

• Among other organs in the body where we find smooth muscles are the urinary bladder, the muscles of the uterus in women, which help to expel the baby at the moment of birth, and in the eye, helping to focus on objects.

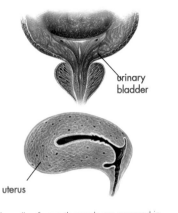

urinary bladder

uterus

The cells of smooth muscle are arranged in layers one above the other.

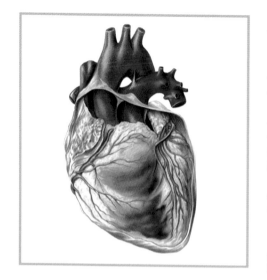

**In heart attacks, part
of the cardiac muscle no
longer receives oxygen
and stops functioning.**

Why do muscles hurt?

The factors that cause painful areas in muscles can be divided into four groups:

• Bad posture, which in general is associated with abnormal postures related to work or with wearing high heels, for example.

• Congenital alterations in the vertebral column or the prolonged immobility of certain people with chronic illnesses who have to lie prostrate in bed, are factors that make some people vulnerable.

• Misusing a muscle or overexerting it with excessive frequency can cause muscular pains or the stiffness we all dread.

• Injuries or blows, like for example, sprains.

• Psychological factors such as anxiety, depression, the frustrations of daily life, or work stress are key factors in the development of muscular pain.

• Illnesses like anemia, reduced glucose levels in the blood, premenstrual syndrome, and menopause cause changes in the energy metabolism of the muscle, favoring the development of painful areas or sectors in different muscles of the body.

Stiffness

• Stiffness is caused by overexertion of the muscles, which makes the fibers that form them rupture, producing an inflammatory reaction in the affected muscle.

• The stiffness is painful because the ruptured cells that make up the damaged fibers release sub-

when observed under a microscope, they seem to be made out of strips. Skeletal muscles are very diverse in size and shape, according to the functions that each one of them has to perform. The largest are located in the back and help to support the bones of the vertebral column and keep the body upright.

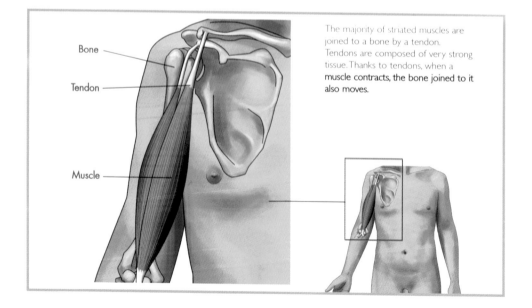

Bone

Tendon

Muscle

The majority of striated muscles are joined to a bone by a tendon. Tendons are composed of very strong tissue. Thanks to tendons, when a **muscle contracts, the bone joined to it also moves.**

> • If pain occurs, consult the doctor so that he can take the necessary steps to diagnose the pain's origin and commence timely and suitable treatment.

stances, such as calcium and potassium, which are irritating and painful.

• To relieve the stiffness and reduce the inflammation, all you need to do is to soak the joint or the injured area in a basin of water with a little ice.

Back pain

• The back is the center of a complex network of nerves, bones, and muscles that work in coordination, so that you can remain upright, move around and relate to the outside world. The back can be schematically divided into two component parts: the vertebral column and the back muscles and ligaments.

• Back pain is a sensation of muscular tension or stiffness, which may or may not be accompanied by pain in the arms or legs.

Advice for avoiding back injuries

Keep good posture.

– It is crucial to keep good posture always.

– Sleep on a firm mattress or place a wooden board between the base of the bed and mattress to provide good support for the back. A mattress that is too soft can cause deviation of the spine. You can sleep on your side with bent knees or lie flat with a pillow under your knees for support.

– Drive with your back against the car seat, close enough to the wheel for your knees to be bent and slightly higher than the hips.

Take physical exercise

– If the back and abdominal muscles are strengthened, this favors correct posture and reduces tension.

– Consult the doctor for his advice as to which exercise is best in each situation.

Control your body weight

– Being overweight, especially in the stomach, causes too much work for the abdominal and back muscles. By reducing body weight, you reduce the need for overexertion and the pain that it can cause. It is advisable to consult a dietician who can plan the optimum diet.

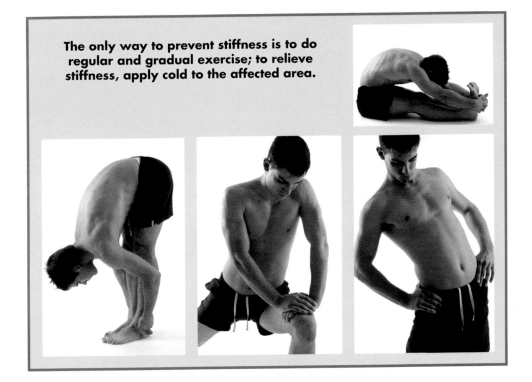

The only way to prevent stiffness is to do regular and gradual exercise; to relieve stiffness, apply cold to the affected area.

PREVENTING BACK INJURIES IS MUCH EASIER THAN CURING THEM

When standing, distribute your weight uniformly.

If you are going to be standing for a long period, **lift one foot onto** a box, or a stair.

When walking, keep your head and shoulders back.

When sitting, keep your back straight leaning against a chair, with **both feet resting on the ground or raised on a footstool, and avoid** sinking into the chair.

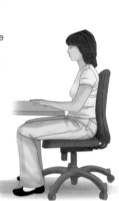

How to lift objects

• Your movements should be slow and smooth. Rapid or violent movements can put excessive strain on your back muscles.

• Keep your body facing the object while lifting. Turning to one side, while lifting the object, can injure your back.

• Keep the load close to your body. Having to raise your arms to lift up and load an object can injure your back.

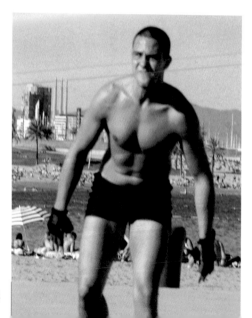

Torticollis

• The muscles, vertebrae, veins, and arteries converge in the neck, which is an anatomical region of special importance. It is an area that must be looked after, particularly to avoid the dreaded affliction known as torticollis.

• Torticollis (which means "rigid neck") is a pathological condition that can be congenital, although in the majority of cases it is acquired, and severe.

Extensive scientific research shows that resting in bed is not an effective treatment for back pain. For example, in support of this, a study demonstrated that a group of patients who rested in bed for a period of two to seven days fared worse than the group who performed the activities that their pain allowed.

To lift something, bend your knees —not your back—to lift the load, keeping your back straight.

• This ailment involves limited neck movement on one side, with the chin pointing towards the other side.

• The neck muscles persistently contract, making the head turn to one side. This type of contraction is called "dystonia" and the muscle associated with torticollis is the sternocleidomastoid.

Common causes of torticollis

The most frequent cause of torticollis is an irritation of the nerves in the neck, which as a secondary effect produces a contraction or a spasm in the neck muscles.

▪ How to treat torticollis

The treatment can include:

• Use of a cervical collar.

• Heat therapy.

• Physiotherapy and massage.

• Ultrasound therapy.

• Drugs.

• Surgery, in case of torticollis at birth.

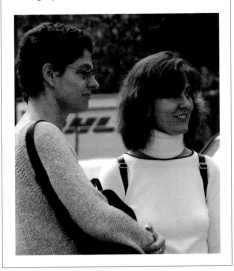

The sternocleidomastoid muscle extends from the sternum to the cranium behind the ear. Torticollis is the result of the shortening of the sternocleidomastoid muscle due to injuries at birth or to incorrect neck posture.

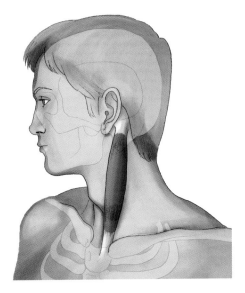

It is a problem that may have different origins: traumatic, inflammatory, postural, etc. Apart from an abrupt movement or an injury, torticollis may be caused by:

• Sleeping in an uncomfortable position.

• Anxiety.

• A muscular injury in the neck at birth.

• A burn.

• Any injury that causes deep scars and shrinkage of the skin.

Muscular spasms of the neck

Torticollis can occur without any known cause (idiopathic), can be of genetic (hereditary), or acquired origin, secondary to injuries of the nervous system, or muscles, and can develop in childhood or adult life.

Torticollis appearing at birth (congenital) may be caused by the head of the fetus being badly positioned in the uterus, by a prenatal injury to the muscles or by blood supply problems in the neck.

How to avoid muscular cramps

- Many muscular pains are due to badly performed exercise and overexertion. Pulled muscles or cramps are frequently caused by lack of warming up before playing sports.

Sports drinks are very effective, since they supply the minerals necessary to prevent cramps and dehydration.

Some advice for preventing cramps

- To be able to control summer cramps, it is best during the hottest months to avoid strenuous physical activities that cause intense sweating. In order to avoid these extremely painful contractions, you must therefore be careful not to be carried away by the summer euphoria and excessive enthusiasm for sports.
- If you swim regularly, do not overexert yourself—cramps in this sport are very frequent, due to the constant stretching involved.
- Magnesium supplements (cocoa, soy, corn, and green vegetables) and potassium (bananas, fresh green vegetables, other vegetables, and dried fruit) are important and help to prevent cramp.
- During cramp or a muscular spasm, it is best to stop your activity, stretch, and massage the painful muscle. At first, heat helps to relax the muscle, although later, the application of ice can act to reduce the pain. If the muscle pain persists, anti-inflammatory non-steroidal medications may be necessary and in more serious cases, antispasmodic medications may be prescribed.

How to treat the pain by means of diet

- It is scientifically proven that the lactovegetarian (fruit and vegetables, milk, and milk products) diet is the healthiest and increases longevity. Within the limits of this diet, there are purifying diets that help to eliminate body toxins. Purifying diets are aimed at drastically eliminating accumulated toxins. However, for this reason, they should be followed for short periods and regulated so as to ensure the body does not become weak.

- With regard to fruit, if it is ripe, in season and consumed in the region where it is produced, it is of high nutritional value, since it is assimilated immediately.
- Another purifying mono-diet is that of whole-grain rice, which is followed for 10 days. Germinated whole grains purify and revitalize the body and can be consumed raw or well cooked in vegetable oil.
- It is a good idea to consult a dietician to find the most suitable diet for each individual.

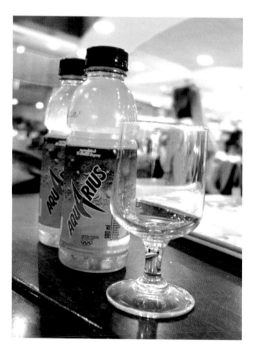

Loss of limbs or other body parts

Loss of limbs or other body parts can be due to injury, illness, or a surgical operation.

Associated symptoms

• Hemorrhage, which can vary in intensity, depending on the location and the cause of the wound.

• The degree of pain does not always seem proportionate to the seriousness of the wound or with the extent of the bleeding.

• In partial loss of limbs, you can observe crushed body tissue, which is torn, although partly attached by muscles, bones, tendons, or skin.

What may cause loss of body parts?

• Loss of body parts is frequently the immediate consequence of accidents in factories and farms with electrical tools or motor vehicles. At home, these accidents may be caused by knife

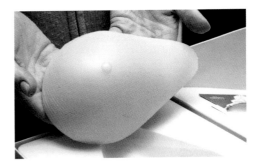

wounds to the fingers or through handling DIY electrical equipment.

• The most serious injuries, especially to the arms, can lead to amputation in 75 percent of cases.

• Certain diseases of the circulatory system, diabetes, blood clots, or osteomyelitis (a bone infection) may require surgical amputation.

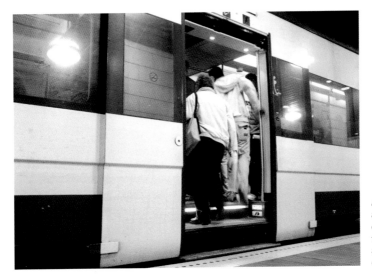

Although it is difficult to be always alert, be particularly careful, especially with anything that can cause an unnecessary accident with serious consequences.

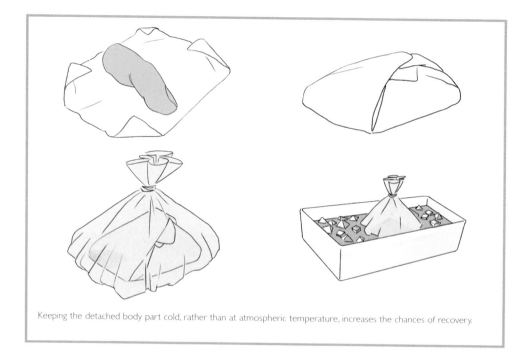

Keeping the detached body part cold, rather than at atmospheric temperature, increases the chances of recovery.

• Lastly, certain surgical operations to extract bone or muscle tumors may involve amputation.

What should be done in the event of injury causing loss of body parts?

If the whole body part is detached:

• First, calm the accident victim down and reassure him. This type of accident is enormously painful and usually terrifies the victim.

• Second, examine the victim's airways to ensure that he is breathing correctly.

• If necessary, carry out cardiopulmonary resuscitation or artificial respiration techniques.

• Try to stop the hemorrhaging, using your hands to exert direct pressure on the wound, raising the injured area, or using pressure points to stop the bleeding.

• If after applying the pressure, the hemorrhaging has not stopped, or if the accident victim has a potentially fatal hemorrhage, try to stop the hemorrhaging, using a bandage that constricts the bleeding area.

• Make the victim lie in a horizontal position and raise his feet about a foot (30 cm).

• Cover him with a blanket or other warm wrapping.

• Do not lay the victim in this position if it is evident that he also has injuries to the head, neck, shoulders, or legs, or if the position proves difficult for him.

• Once you have controlled the hemorrhaging in the place where the body part has been lost, examine the victim to check if there are other

▪ What not to do when a body part is lost

• Do not give the victim anything to drink, especially alcohol, tea, or coffee.

• Do not touch or handle the detached or injured limb.

• Do not try to attach the separated parts.

• Do not make a tourniquet, since this is a very dangerous procedure, risking cardiac arrest when removed. A tourniquet is only used in cases where the hemorrhaging is very severe and there is a high risk of death. Furthermore, it could endanger the whole limb.

signs of injury that need emergency treatment. Fractures, cuts, or other injuries must be treated appropriately.

• It is very important to remain at the victim's side until medical assistance arrives.

What to do with the detached body part:

• The body part that has become detached, should be wrapped in sterile moist gauze, placed in a plastic bag that can be sealed and submerged in a bucket containing water and ice or, failing that, in cold water.

• The detached body part must reach the surgeon as quickly as possible, given that with the passage of time the chances of re-attaching it diminish.

• By subjecting the detached part to a temperature of some 40°F (4°C), which is the temperature achievable with ice and water, it can be maintained in conditions suitable for re-attachment for about 18 hours, if not, this procedure will only be possible for 4 to 6 hours.

• When delivering the detached limb to the emergency medical team, you must inform them as to how it became severed, whether it was cut off cleanly, ripped off, or crushed.

If the body part is partially detached:

• In the case of a limb or other body part becoming partially or incompletely detached, do not pull off or separate it, respecting any physical connection, however small.

• The same procedures should be carried out as in the case of complete loss of body parts, but in this instance, you should try to keep the limb in place, immobilizing it.

• It is essential not to hurt or damage the tissue joining the two separated parts, or to poke in the wound. Although these types of physical connections may be weak, it is very important to conserve them.

• Under no circumstances should the detached limb be separated from the body when some tissue remains. In fact, you should do the opposite: keep each part in contact with the other, although without trying to reconnect them.

People who have suffered this type of accident are advised to go for rehabilitation to learn how to control the complications, such as "phantom pain,"—that is to say, the sensation of pain that appears where the missing body part used to be.

• In the case of complete loss of body parts (the body part has become completely detached), caused by a blow or accident, it is sometimes possible to reattach the part, especially if the stump and the detached part have received the necessary care.

• In the case of complete loss of body parts, depending on the severity of the injury, some connective tissue will remain, thus making it possible to join the two parts together again.

• However, you must take into account other factors that may affect the recovery of the injury, such as possible infections and severe hemorrhaging.

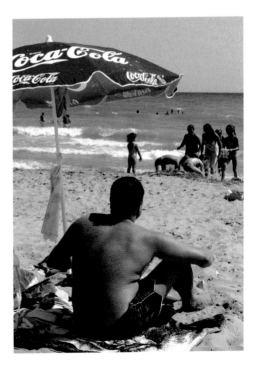

Glue adhesions

The newest adhesives and glues, containing cyanoacrylate (superglue), must be used with great caution, since a moment of carelessness can lead to adhesion of the skin. Certain safety rules should be followed to avoid little accidents that can cause skin lesions and wounds. In case of doubt, get the necessary information from a toxicology center.

What are they?

• Glues, adhesives, and resins are substances capable of joining materials together by physical or chemical means.

• They usually have different components, the most common being the following:

– Cyanoacrylates.
– Contact adhesives.
– Polyurethane.
– Acrylics.
– In the home, they are used to stick things together.

Preventing glue adhesions

• A series of steps should be followed to avoid contact with, or poisoning by the glue while handling it:

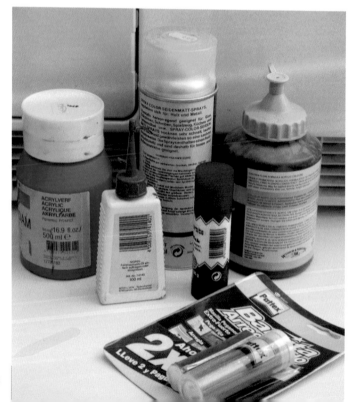

Before using any glue, read the safety instructions that come with it.

Effects of glue adhesion

- Generally, though depending on the type of glue that has adhered to you, there will be irritation to the skin, the mucus linings of the eyes, and the respiratory system.
- Rapid-action glues cause burns to the skin through contact alone.
- If the glue has come into contact with a considerable area of skin, the burns can be serious.

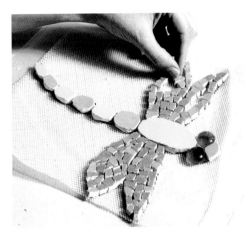

– If you are going to use the glue for a prolonged period, for example when doing handwork requiring the use of adhesives, resins, and solvents, keep the room where you are working well ventilated. If it is not possible to ventilate the room, you should protect yourself by means of masks and extractors.

– If you are going to do handwork requiring frequent use of glue, you should also use eye protection.

– When using these types of glue, you should protect your hands with gloves, to avoid direct contact with the skin. It is also advisable to wear old clothing, since glue can also damage textiles.

– If gloves are not available, you can use a protective cream, whose function is to create a barrier between the skin and the glue. This cream should be applied as often as necessary when you are using the glue. The protective cream must be applied after washing your hands with soap and water.

– When working with glue, keep it away from food and drink, since they may become contaminated.

– Given that this type of glue is inflammable, it is also important to keep it away from any heat source or from things or objects that can cause sparks or flames.

– Following on from the previous point, it is important not to smoke when using glue, or to use lighters or matches.

On most occasions, it is possible to separate the affected parts of your body. Generally, the eyelids become unstuck by themselves in about one to four days.

What to do in the case of glue adhesion

If the glue sticks to you, follow the steps below:

- Put the affected area immediately under hot water, dry it carefully, and apply moisturizing cream.
- If the glue has fallen on your eyelids, try to keep them unstuck. If this is not possible and they are glued, call emergency medical services immediately. Do not try to free your eyelids by yourself, since this involves a very delicate operation that can only be performed by health professionals. In any case, when your sweat starts to accumulate, this may possibly cause the eyelids to free themselves without external help.
- If the glue has got directly into your eyes, wash them out thoroughly for 10 minutes, keeping them under the faucet with your eyelids open. If the irri-

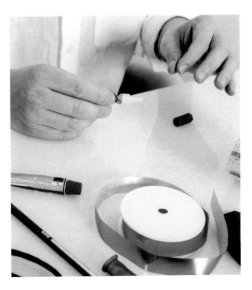

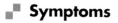

Symptoms

Respiratory
- Breathing difficulties due to inhalation.
- Inflammation of the throat, which can also cause respiratory problems.

Eyes, ears, nose, and throat
- Severe pain in the throat.
- Severe pain or burning in the nose, eyes, ears, lips, or tongue.
- Loss of vision.

Gastrointestinal
- Intense abdominal pain.
- Vomiting.
- Burns in the esophagus.
- Vomiting with blood.
- Blood in the feces.

Blood
- Severe changes in the acidity levels in the blood that can damage all the body organs.

Skin
- Irritation.
- Burning.
- Necrosis (death) of the skin and underlying tissue.

Cardiovascular
- Rapid development of hypotension
- Collapse.

tation continues or gives you pain, see an ophthalmologist.
- If one finger has become glued to another, try to separate them by making very gentle circular movements, taking care not to tear the skin. If this yields no result, use acetone, if you have some at home. But never use acetone on your eyes, mouth, or tongue.
- If your clothing is impregnated with glue, take it off quickly to avoid the risk of it sticking to your skin.

- If the glue is on a small area of skin which is not around the eyes or mouth, it is not necessary to remove it, since the skin can stretch to accommodate it. In this case, wash the area with soap and hot water, and use a flat narrow object, not a pointed one—for example, the handle of a spoon—to gently remove the remains of the glue that is still attached.

What should be done?
With this type of poisoning, you must seek immediate medical assistance. It is important:
- Not to induce vomiting.
- If the eyes or skin have been exposed, to wash them well and bathe your eyes with water.
- If you have ingested the product, drink water to dilute it.

Domestic glue is relatively nontoxic in small quantities; however, the inhalation or ingestion of any quantity by a small child can be dangerous.

Respect the safety rules

- Adhesives are inflammable and toxic substances, and should therefore be kept away from heat and out of the reach of young children. After using them, close the container hermetically.

- Avoid inhaling these products. Some of them can cause irritation, like cyanoacrylate or hard plastic adhesive.

- Apply it very carefully avoiding contact with the skin. Extreme care should be taken in the case of cyanoacrylate. Disposable gloves may be used for protection.

- On no account touch the colored nozzle of a spray gun or the recently applied adhesive, since this causes burns. Keep the spray gun upright, visible, and away from possible contact.

Traffic accidents

In a traffic accident, the treatment of injuries should be left in the hands of the professionals. However, any driver can stop in order to warn others of the accident and provide first aid assistance.

Traffic accidents

• If you witness a traffic accident, you must call the highway emergency medical services, so that they can come urgently. A series of steps can be followed to prepare the accident site before they arrive.

Do not light matches or smoke in the vicinity of the accident vehicle, because of the danger of the car exploding.

• Do not feel that you are obliged to help in a dangerous situation or to intervene in an accident in a impulsive manner without knowing the steps to follow.

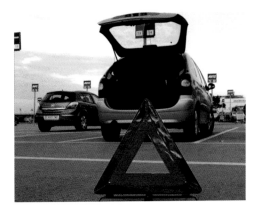

Emergency triangles should be placed at a distance of approximately 150 yards (140 meters) from the accident vehicle.

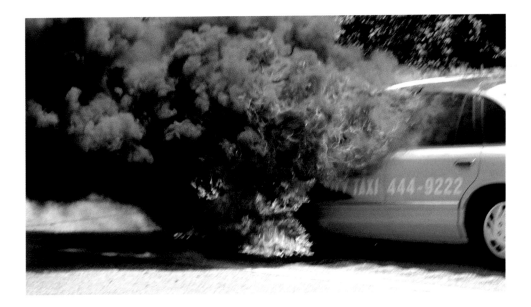

Three people assisting an accident victim.

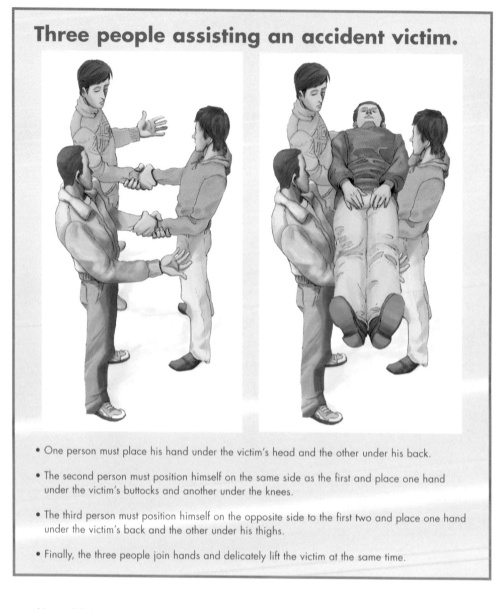

- One person must place his hand under the victim's head and the other under his back.

- The second person must position himself on the same side as the first and place one hand under the victim's buttocks and another under the knees.

- The third person must position himself on the opposite side to the first two and place one hand under the victim's back and the other under his thighs.

- Finally, the three people join hands and delicately lift the victim at the same time.

- Above all, it is very important to remain calm and collected at every moment.
- Keep your vehicle's emergency lights on. If possible, park behind the accident vehicle and some distance from it, in a safe position.
- Place emergency warning triangles in appropriate places to warn approaching vehicles. On getting out of your car, proceed with care, so as not to be run down by other vehicles.
- If possible, stop the motor of the accident vehicle, turning off the ignition or disconnecting the battery. Secure the car with the parking brake.
- If there has been an oil or gasoline spillage, indicate this and throw earth or sand over it, never water.
- Do not smoke or light matches around the accident site.
- If the victim is a motorcyclist, as a general rule, do not remove his helmet.
- Loosen the victim's clothing, to prevent it constricting him and aggravating possible injuries.

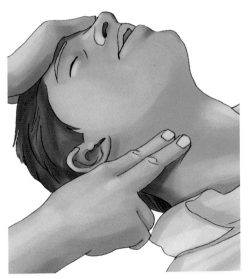

Checking the pulse from the carotid artery

What to do in the case of spinal injury

- Do not under any circumstances move the casualty; this will aggravate the state of the injury if incorrect movements are made.
- Only in the case of vomiting should the victim's head be gently turned to one side.
- If the victim is a motorcyclist, do not remove his helmet, or allow anyone else to do so. This rule has only one exception, which is in the case of cardio-respiratory arrest—if the victim is not breathing, has no pulse, and the type of helmet does not permit you to perform resuscitation techniques.

— Do not touch or move those who are injured. This should be left in the hands of the emergency specialists. Only move the injured if you suspect that the vehicle is about to catch fire, explode, or fall into the water. If there is a fire, use the extinguisher or extinguishers of the vehicles involved or blankets, earth, or sand, but never water.

— The safest way to move a victim is with several people together, as though transporting a rigid mass. Never move an injured casualty when there is only one person who can offer assistance.

When you call the emergency services, give them the following information:

- The name of the person who is phoning.
- The telephone number of the phone you are using.
- The exact location of the accident, the road, and the mileage distance.
- The number of victims and an assessment of their injuries.
- The number of vehicles involved in the accident and their type, whether they are cars, trucks, buses or motorcycles.
- The weather conditions of the area (if it is raining or snowing, if it is windy, etc.).
- If there has been a spillage of gasoline, oil, or other liquids at risk of exploding or catching fire.

How to move accident victims

- Proceed in the following way:
- It is advisable to place the victim flat on his back, with his extended arms resting against his trunk, his palms facing upwards, and his legs also extended.
- The people assisting should kneel on each side of the accident victim.
- If an injured person has remained lying in an area of the road where he is in danger, drag him away by his feet, never his arms.

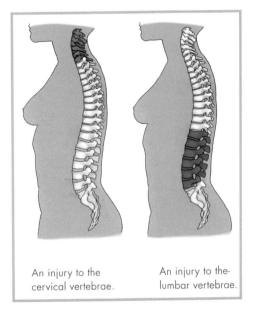

An injury to the cervical vertebrae.

An injury to the-lumbar vertebrae.

The state of shock

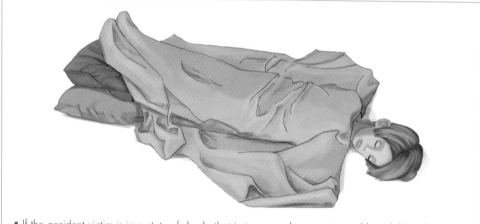

- If the accident victim is in a state of shock, that is to say, pale, sweating, cold, and the pulse is weak and fast, you should raise his legs, cover him with a blanket, and move his head to one side if no neck injury is suspected.

– If the injured person is lying in an area of the road where he is in no danger, but is bleeding from the face or vomiting, or is unconscious, place him on his side without twisting his body.

Assessing the injuries

- You must assess all the injured people as quickly as possible and begin to assist those who are in the most serious condition.
- Assess the vital functions of the victim.
- Check if the casualty is conscious, by trying to speak to him and seeing if he replies, touching and pinching him to see if he reacts to stimulus. If the victim is unconscious, undo the buttons of his clothing and release his seat belt.
- Check if the victim is breathing. To do this, you have to get up close to his nose or mouth, and see if you can hear any breathing. You can also check if any air is coming out of his nostrils by placing the back of your hand under them.
- Check the pulse. This is done by placing your hand on the carotid artery.
- If the casualty has stopped breathing, but has a pulse, you should do mouth-to-mouth resuscitation.

In the event of bleeding:

- If there are bleeding wounds, use a sterile bandage or a cloth or clean white fabric, with the aim of putting pressure on the wound and trying to stop the bleeding.

- Maintain the pressure for several minutes.
- If bandages of a compress type are available, place them over the wound and exert pressure on it.
- If the bandages or dressings used to contain the bleeding become soaked, it is not advisable to change them for new bandages; you need only place dry and clean bandages over those that are already soaked in blood.

If you suspect that a person has a spinal injury

- This type of injury is very delicate, since if the vertebrae are affected, this can damage the spinal medulla, causing different types of injuries of a very serious nature, depending on how high up the spinal column they are.
  – Quadriplegia: the spinal injuries are located at the neck, causing paralysis and loss of feeling in the arms and legs.
  – Paraplegia: the spinal injuries are located at the level of the thoracic or lumbar vertebrae, causing paralysis and loss of feeling in the legs.
- Fractures to the vertebral column occur because of abrupt movement of the spine due to the accident (for example, when the vehicle stops suddenly or after an impact from the rear), with the head hitting against the windshield or the ground in accidents with two-wheeled vehicles, and in cases where the occupants or the driver are thrown out of the vehicle.

What to do in the case of head and neck injuries

- Place sterile dressings or bandages over the wounds and wait for the emergency services.
- Bleeding from the ears or nose should be stemmed with plugs.
- Check the victim's breathing, pulse, and state of consciousness.
- Check for any possible obstacles to breathing, such as blood, secretions, and other foreign bodies.
- Do not move the victim in any event, especially if he is unconscious.

• If the traumatism is sufficiently severe to damage the structure of the vertebrae, it can be accompanied by injury to the spinal medulla that lies inside the vertebrae.
• There may be spinal injuries:
– If the victim is unconscious.
– If there are injuries or blows to the head.
– If the victim is a motorcyclist.
– If the victim is conscious, but evidently cannot move his arms and/or his legs.

When to suspect head or neck injuries
• If the victim is unconscious.

What to do in the case of injuries to the chest and abdomen

- First, follow the general advice: protect the accident victim, place warning signs at the accident site, and call the emergency services.
- If the victim is conscious and not vomiting, try to make him to sit up gently, since this type of injury is often associated with breathing difficulties.
- If the injury is open, do not poke in the wound, or try to put the organs back in place. If sterile bandages are available, place them over the area for protection.

• If there is bleeding from the ears and nose (this can signify that the victim has suffered a cranial fracture).
• Superficial injuries to the head or neck may indicate more serious injury.

Injuries to the chest and abdomen
• These types of injuries are very serious and on many occasions endanger the casualty's life. In general, it is advisable to wait for the arrival of the emergency medical services, who will be responsi-

▪ Advice for avoiding traffic accidents

- Respect the recommended safe distance.
- Drive at a prudent speed when negotiating bends, and when driving on a wet or slippery road; avoid braking sharply.
- Do not consume alcohol if you are going to drive.
- Make a rest stop every two hours or every 100 miles (160 kilometers) to prevent fatigue.
- Do not exceed the maximum speed limits.

- Choose vehicles equipped with ABS, which provide better stability in case of braking sharply. On braking sharply, press the clutch pedal at the same time as the brake pedal. By doing this, all the braking power is harnessed to stop the vehicle.
- If you judge that you will not have time to brake, try to avoid whatever you are going to collide with. This maneuver should be carried out with your hands on the steering wheel the whole time.

First aid courses

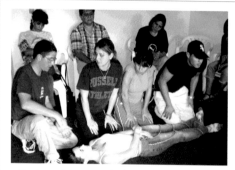

• Find out if there are highway first aid courses being offered in your area. It is usually basic training, but very useful and may save lives if at some time you have to treat people injured in a road accident.

• Assistance during the first minutes of a traffic accident could be crucial for saving many lives.

• According to Red Cross statistics, 57 percent of deaths occur in the minutes following an accident at the site itself, and of this percentage, 85 percent of deaths are due to the obstruction of the victim's airways, which could have been avoided with simple resuscitation procedures.

ble for carrying out appropriate assistance procedures.

• Chest and abdominal injuries tend to be caused by hitting against the steering wheel or other parts of the car, or through not using a seat belt or using it incorrectly.

• Blows to the chest and abdomen can be divided into two types: the closed type, if the skin tissue has not been torn, or the open type, when the skin tissue has been torn and has bleeding wounds.

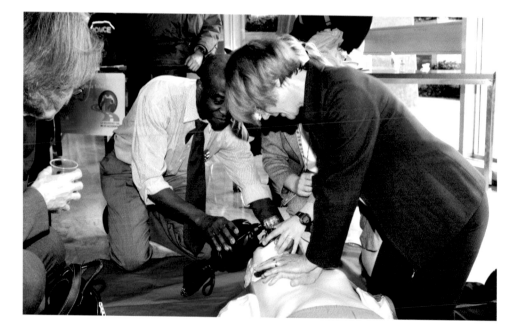

Stings

Normally, insects do not sting humans unless they feel that their habitat is being invaded, or if they feel threatened. It is important to keep the area of the bite very clean to avoid subsequent infections, since insects are often carriers of pathogens.

Stings

• Stings are defined as injuries that first affect the body's soft tissue, but which, according to the progress and response of each person, can endanger life, and even cause death if the injury is not treated correctly and rapidly, especially with people who suffer serious allergic reactions.

• Insects, arthropods, and marine animals can attack human beings with stings that inflict small puncture wounds. They often inject toxic substances, which can act locally or throughout the body, depending on the animal that has caused the sting and the quantity of toxin injected.

Stings of flying insects and ants
• The oral structure of wasps and ants is for

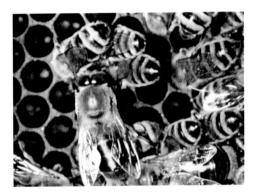

Stings have one complication: the infections caused by the germs injected during the bite, such as the tetanus infection.

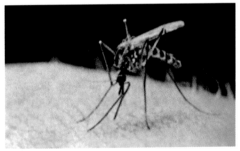

When to go to the doctor

• If the inflammation and redness extend beyond the area of the sting.

• If the area appears infected or festers.

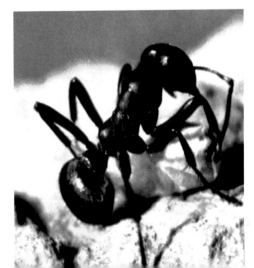

■ General considerations

The following general care should be given when someone has been stung by an insect:

- Wash the area of the sting with soap and water.
- If there is bleeding, try to stop it by exerting pressure on the sting for several minutes.
- Cover the sting with a sterile dressing.
- Other factors affect the severity of a sting:
  - If the sting is multiple or is on the face and/or the neck, where it is usually more serious.

- If the insect has stung the victim inside the mouth, this can cause inflammation of the mucus linings and difficulty in breathing.
- If the individual who has been stung is allergic to insect stings, this can cause anaphylactic shock.
- If the victim is a baby, a young child, or an elderly person, the situation is more serious.

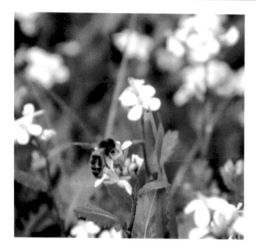

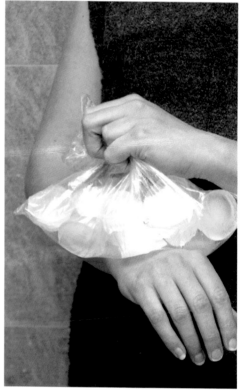

masticating in general, and in bees it is for masticating and licking, and their means of defense, in most species, is f a sting.

- In the case of mosquitoes, specifically in the female mosquito, they use their oral apparatus to pierce the skin and suck the blood of animals, including humans. While they suck the blood, they can transmit diseases that they carry.

What can cause an insect sting

- Insects tend to feel threatened and disturbed in the presence of strong smells, for example cologne, perfume, or sweat.
- Abrupt movements also disturb them, which is why it is advisable to stay still when an insect approaches until it goes away.
- Strong winds that may shake their hive also make them feel threatened; so you should not

Insects' stings are usually located in the abdomen and contain toxic substances.

shake or hit the hives or nests of bees, since you risk being stung by a swarm.

• After being stung by a scorpion, there is usually:
– Intense pain in the area.
– Local inflammation.
– The skin changes color in the area of the sting, normally turning a lighter color.

In the event of a scorpion sting, take care to do the following:

• Apply an ice pack over the area of the sting to soothe the inflammation and reduce the pain and absorption of the poison.

• Leave the ice pack on for about ten minutes, take it off for another ten minutes, and repeat the operation until the inflammation goes down.

• Keep the victim motionless.

Bites from spiders and ticks

During the process of sucking blood, ticks penetrate the skin with part of their body in a parasitic way, which is why you have to be very careful when removing them.

The symptoms of spider and tick bites are usually:
• Intense pain in the area.
• Local inflammation.
• The skin changes color in the area of the sting, normally acquiring a reddish color.
• In the case of spiders, you can sometimes see two red dots in the area of the bite.

Ticks feed on the blood of mammals, including humans. These creatures live on the skin of animals parasitically.

How to remove ticks

• The best way to remove a tick is when it is already dead. To kill it, you need to use insecticide products, and then with latex gloves and tweezers you can carefully remove it without breaking its skin. It is advisable not to squeeze or squash the tick, because this can lead to bacterial infection.

• Once the tick has been removed from the skin, disinfect the wound. Wash the skin by rubbing it with soap and water, to eliminate the pathogens that have remained in the wound.

• Rest the affected area.

• If the tick cannot be removed, take the victim to the emergency room—if part of the tick remains inside the skin, it can lead to infection.

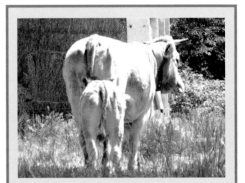

To avoid tick bites, it is best not to walk through fields where cattle are grazing, since they are often plagued by ticks.

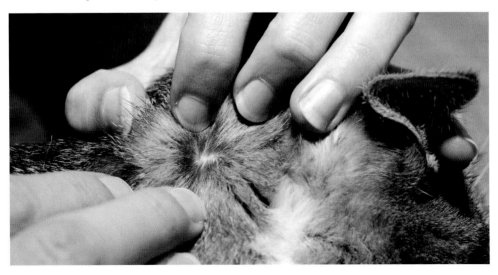

An black widow spider with a globe-shaped body and characteristic red patches.

The black widow is thus named because of its dark color and the fact that it devours the male after copulation. This spider is found in warm, humid, rural areas in North America. It is usually found outdoors, but also in dark, quiet places, like cellars. This spider's sting does not generally endanger life, except in the case of young children and the elderly, but causes very painful muscular contractions, especially in the abdominal area. It also causes severe sweating.

▪ What should be done in the case of a spider bite?

- You should apply an ice pack over the area of the bite to soothe the inflammation and reduce the pain and absorption of the poison.
- Leave the ice pack on for about ten minutes, take it off for another ten minutes, and repeat the operation until the inflammation goes down.
- The victim should remain motionless.

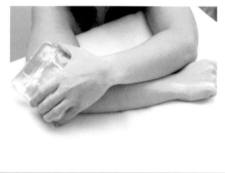

▪ What should you do when bitten by a black widow?

- Go to the emergency room and tell them about the bite. The doctor will prescribe medications that reduce the pain caused by the bite and muscular relaxants for the abdominal contractions.

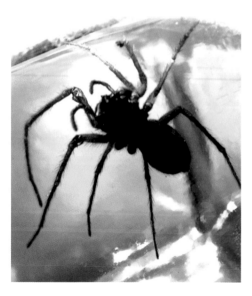

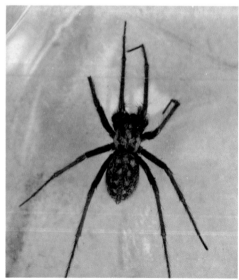

Bites

If the skin is broken, animal bites can cause infections and transmit diseases such as rabies. The extent of the bite depends on the size of the animal concerned. Snakes are normally peaceful animals that do not bite unless they feel threatened. The severity of the bite depends on whether the creature has injected poison and on the sensitivity of the victim to that particular venom.

Different kinds of bites

Dog bites

• Ninety percent of animal bites are caused by dogs.

• Dog bites and scratches even when light, can infect and spread bacteria to other parts of the body. All dogs can transmit diseases when they bite, especially rabies.

• Children under ten years old are the most common victims. In most cases, the bite occurs because the victim has upset the dog.

• The larger a dog is, the greater the size of its bite. The severity of a dog bite can vary from a simple scratch to tearing of the flesh, with the bleeding that results. The areas most frequently injured are usually the extremities of the body.

• When you go to the medical center, you should have the following information and do what is suggested below:

Dogs should not be allowed outdoors without a lead and muzzle. If your neighbors have dogs, you should ask them to control their dogs and not to let them loose.

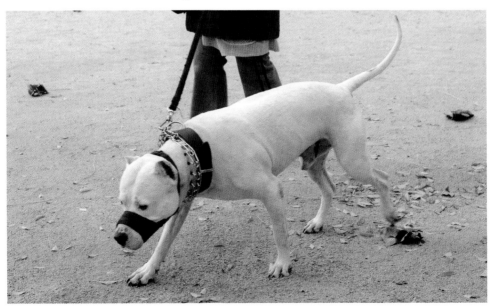

▪ What should be done in the case of a dog bite?

- Drive the animal away with a stick or by waving some other large object and shouting.
- Clean the superficial wounds with soap and water and apply antiseptic. If you have latex gloves to hand, use them for protection against exposure to the other person's blood.
- Cover the serious wounds and put pressure on the bleeding with sterile gauze.
- Take the victim to a medical center, so that the doctor can decide if it is necessary to give him a vaccination. When an individual is bitten by an animal, he will probably have to take antibiotics, receive an anti-tetanus booster vaccine, or the anti-rabies vaccine. Bites and scratches on the hands or face of a child are especially prone to infection and should be examined by a doctor.

• Secure the dog that caused the attack and find out if possible if it is vaccinated against rabies. It is especially important to secure a stray dog.

• If it is known that the dog is vaccinated against rabies, ask when it had its last anti-rabies vaccination.

• Inform the doctor of any unusual behavior in the dog, in case there is a chance that it has rabies.

• Help to control the dog, if it is obedient.

• If a child is involved, bring his vaccination card.

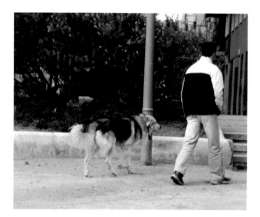

Children must be taught to treat dogs correctly, without ever upsetting them, especially when they are eating or asleep.

Preventing dog bites

• The majority of dog bites can be prevented, since they generally occur because children upset the dogs concerned.

• You should always watch over children when they are near dogs. Prevent the child approaching strange dogs. Never leave a child alone with a dog.

• Never stroke a dog without first letting him sniff you.

• Children should also be taught not to approach stray dogs or feed them.

• It is not advisable to approach an animal that might have rabies, or to try to capture it by yourself.

• If you have a dog at home, it should be vaccinated regularly and you should ask your friends and acquaintances to do the same with their dogs.

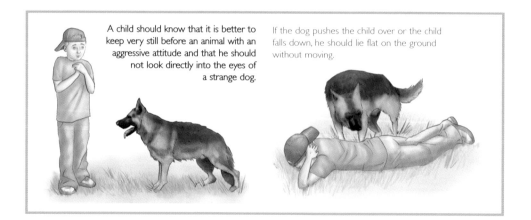

A child should know that it is better to keep very still before an animal with an aggressive attitude and that he should not look directly into the eyes of a strange dog.

If the dog pushes the child over or the child falls down, he should lie flat on the ground without moving.

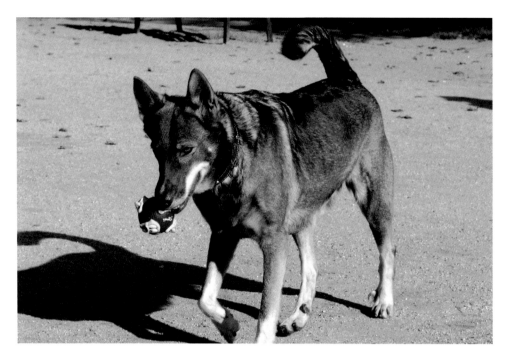

Advice about choosing a dog for a pet

• It is important to take your time in choosing the breed of dog that most suits your needs. To do this, you should consult a veterinarian and read books about different breeds.

• Do not buy a dog because you like the way it looks.

• If you have small children in the house, it is best to get a puppy.

• If you have a baby in the house, check the dog's vaccination timetable carefully to eliminate any possible risk of infection.

• Aggressive breeds of dogs are not suitable for families with children.

• Castrated males are generally less aggressive.

Cat bites

• Cat bites are much less frequent than dog bites, but they can end up being more dangerous.

• Unlike dogs, cats do not cause tearing wounds, but with their pointed teeth, inflict deep wounds which constitute a greater risk of infection.

• A cat scratch can transmit a bacterial infection, even when the scratch does not seem to be infected.

• If cat bites infect your system, this can cause redness, swelling around the wound, swelling of the lymph glands, fever, sweating, shivering, and cramps, etc.

If possible, it is advisable to take a dog to a training school. This will reduce the risks to the family and the people who come into contact with it.

▪ What should be done in the case of a cat bite?

• Clean the superficial wounds with soap and water and apply antiseptic. If there are latex gloves available, use them for protection against exposure to the other person's blood.

• Cover the serious wounds and put pressure on the bleeding with sterile gauze.

• Take the victim to a medical center, so that the doctor can decide if it is necessary to give him a vaccination. When a person is bitten by an animal, he will probably have to take antibiotics, receive an anti-tetanus booster vaccine or the anti-rabies vaccine. Bites and scratches on the hands or face of a child are especially prone to infection and should be examined by a doctor.

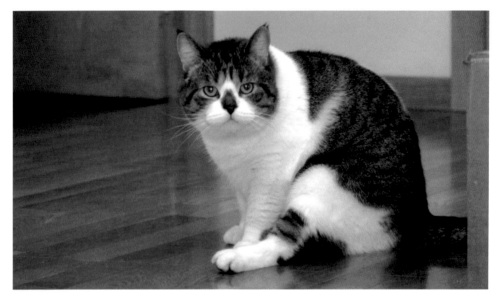

Anti-rabies vaccine

The anti-rabies vaccine for some years now has been reserved for professionals, such as veterinarians, laboratory personnel, and slaughterhouse workers, etc, who habitually come into contact with animals. The anti-rabies vaccine is recommended for all travelers above the age of one.

The vaccine that is currently administered is very effective against the disease, which is very serious and can cause death. Given that animal bites are inevitable, it is very important for domestic animals also to be vaccinated.

Cats should also be vaccinated against rabies, even if they do not leave the house.

Snakebites

• Snakebites are one of the most frequent and dangerous accidents that happen in the countryside.

• Snakes are generally peaceful animals and nonaggressive, and take flight when they hear a noise. They only attack when they feel threat-

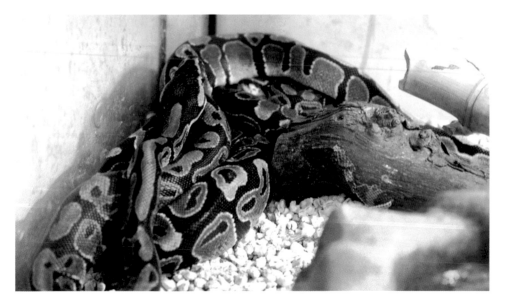

What should be done in the case of a snakebite?

- Get away as quickly as possible from the snake that has bitten you. Snakes normally disappear quickly, but there is always a chance of another bite, and subsequent bites normally inject more poison than the first.

- Try to calm the nervous state of the individual who has been bitten.

- Make him lie on the ground and try to stop him moving, to prevent the blood circulation increasing the absorption of the poison.

- Wash the wound with soap and water.

- Apply ice.

- If the bite has occurred on an extremity, try to immobilize it.

- Take off rings or any other object that constricts, since the affected area may swell.

- Take the victim to the emergency room.

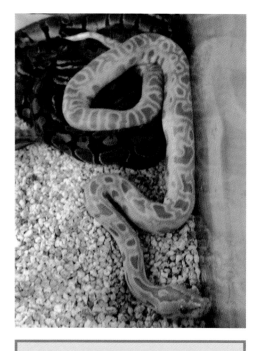

It is not advisable to suck out the poison with your mouth, since there may be small lesions or cuts inside your mouth and these might become affected by the same poison.

ened or when someone gets in their way. Their bites normally cause wounds and should therefore be treated in a similar way. The majority of snakes bite the extremities of the body.

- It is often very difficult to know what species of snake has attacked the victim, since they tend to get away from the site where the bite occurred.

Preventing snakebites

- If you are walking through the countryside, wear thick pants and shoes that protect your feet, like ankle boots or high boots.

- If you are walking at night, it is better to take a good flashlight. The majority of snakes are nocturnal.

Symptoms caused by snakebites

Snakebites usually produce the following symptoms:
- Inflammation in the area of the bite.
- Intense pain.
- If the snake that has bitten you is poisonous, the symptoms are aggravated and may include the following:
  - A state of shock.
  - Anxiety.
  - Nausea and vomiting.
  - Convulsions.
  - Coma.
- The severity of snakebites depends on factors such as:
  - The age and height of the victim.
  - The location of the bite.
  - The number of bites.
  - The quantity of venom injected.
  - The sensitivity of the victim to the venom.

There are 3,000 species of snakes in the whole world, but only ten percent are venomous.

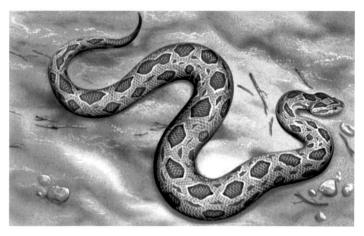

• Be careful when lifting rocks in case there is a snake underneath.

• If you come face to face with a snake, the best thing is not to disturb it and get away from there immediately.

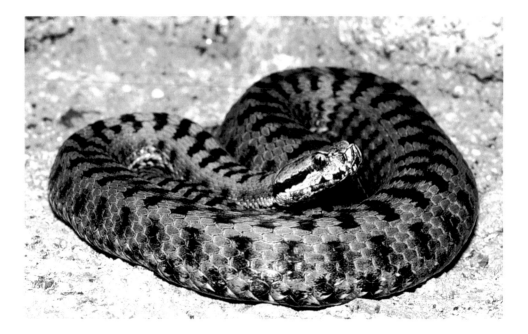

Allergies while on vacation

Allergies are disproportionate reactions of the body to allergens. Among the most common allergens are pollen, mites, some animals, foods, and certain medications. Allergies can cause illnesses, such as allergic rhinitis or asthma. While on vacation, you can reduce allergic attacks by following certain recommended steps.

In the car

- Cars tend to be full of common allergens, such as dust mites and mold spores.

- The mites are usually to be found in the carpets of the vehicle, in the upholstery, and the ventilation filters.

- Before setting out on a long car journey, it is advisable to put on the heater or the air-conditioning with the vehicle windows wide open for about ten minutes; in this way you eliminate the mites and mold spores that may have collected in the ventilation system.

- However, these common allergens are also to be found outside, so if you are allergic to dust mites or mold spores, it is advisable to get anti-pollen filters for the car and to travel with the windows shut and the air-conditioning on.

- When traveling by car, you should go during the early morning or at night, when air quality is better and so it is less dangerous for the allergy sufferer.

- Do not allow smoking in the car, since cigarette smoke can make the allergy sufferer's condition worse.

Allergies while on vacation

Allergies can affect you on vacation and when traveling. You can prevent these attacks by following certain cautionary advice, and so avoid the chance of your leisure time being spoiled and make traveling more pleasant.

Clean your car frequently and use a powerful vacuum cleaner to eliminate dust mites and other allergens.

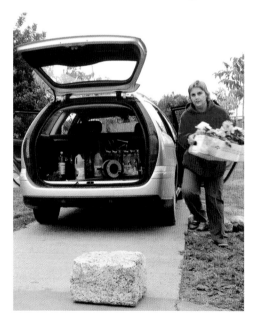

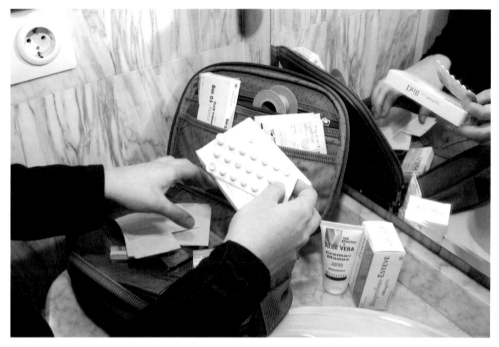

It is best to keep medications in your hand luggage, to use in case of need and so you do not lose them if the baggage goes astray.

• Before going on vacation, you should find out about changes in climate and temperature of the place you are visiting and go to the doctor for information about the precautions you need to take.

• Allergens such as dust mites, mold spores, and pollen float in the air.

• Individuals allergic to insect bites should take the appropriate drugs with them in case they are bitten.

On the airplane

• If the allergy sufferer has severe bronchial asthma, it is possible that when the airplane reaches an altitude of approximately 30,000 feet (9,000 m), he may need additional supplies of oxygen. In this case, it is necessary to warn the airline well in advance of taking the flight. The company cannot under any circumstances deny your right to travel with extra oxygen supplies.

The climate

• Exposure to allergens and irritating substances varies according to climate, temperature, and season.

• When traveling to the tropics, the climate is humid and warm, exposing you more to allergens, such as mites and mold spores circulating in the air and pollen from the vegetation typical of that region.

• When traveling to cold and humid climates, you are more exposed to dust mites and mold spores inside houses.

• When traveling to dry and cold climates, asthmatics may suffer irritation to their airways and therefore be more prone to breating difficulties.

• The general advice is to avoid vacations in places with humid climates. It is necessary to get comprehensive information about the area you are going to visit, given that there are certain microclimates that may trigger allergic attacks.

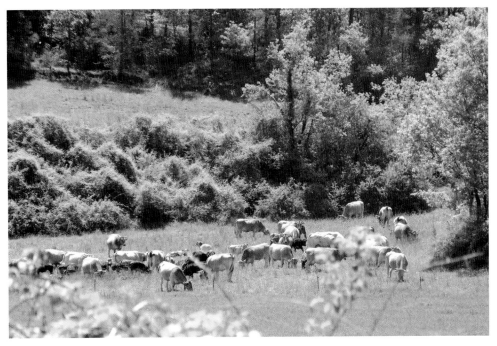

It is best for allergy sufferers to vacation in areas having warm, dry, and sunny climates with little wind.

• If you are allergic to foods, be careful about food on the plane. When you ask the airline company staff, they cannot tell you the exact ingredients of the food, since food on planes is usually provided by an independent catering company. In that case, it is advisable to take your own food from home and, if this is not possible, take medication to use in case of a severe reaction to the food.

• If the allergy causes infections in the ears or nose, such as sinusitis, these ailments may get worse. It is best to delay the flight until the symptoms have improved somewhat, or to go to an allergy specialist who may prescribe a decongestant. To avoid earache during the flight, it is helpful to chew gum, yawn, and drink a lot of liquid.

If you are not used to playing sports in the mountains, ask the doctor to recommend the kind of physical activity most suitable for you. The doctor may possibly carry out a physical examination before you go on vacation.

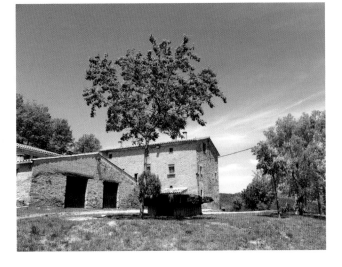

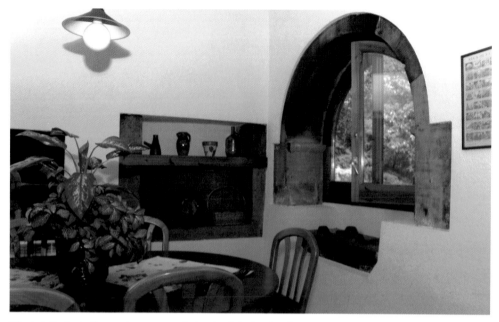

If the hotel is situated in a rural area or near the beach, ask the hotel staff to air and clean the room thoroughly before you arrive.

• If the allergy causes rhinitis and the nasal passages are irritated, this condition may get worse during a plane trip, since the air in planes has very low humidity and may dry out the nasal passages. In this case, you should consult the pharmacist so that he can prescribe nasal sprays that help to maintain the nasal passages at their correct level of humidity.

• Take a sufficient quantity of medication for the whole journey and keep it in its original package so that it can be duly identified if required by customs officials.

• In some countries they spray airplane cabins with insecticide after the plane has landed and while the passengers are still on board. They do

In the hotel

- In hotels, the concentration of allergens, such as dust mites and mold spores tends to be quite high.

- They are usually to be found on the mattresses, carpets, and upholstered armchairs.

- The cleaning products that are used in hotels can also irritate the mucus membranes of people who are more sensitive to these products.

- Before reserving a hotel room, it is advisable to ask if rooms are available for people with allergies.

- If people are allergic to mold spores, they should request a sunny, dry room that is far from swimming pools, gymnasiums, or other damp areas.

- If you are allergic to animals, ask the hotel staff what the rules are regarding the admission of pets and reserve a room where animals have not been permitted.

- Do not allow people free access to the room.

- If an individual is allergic to dust mites, he can bring anti-allergic undersheets and pillow-cases and even bed linen if the symptoms are frequently severe.

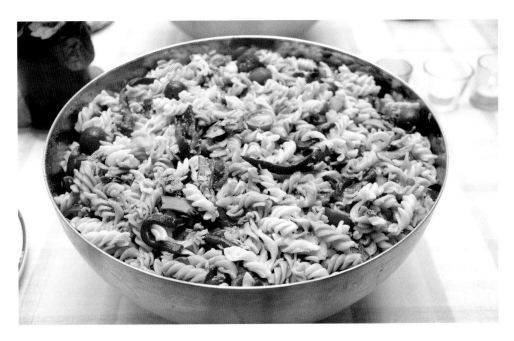

this to avoid the entry of mosquitoes and other insects that might bring infestations from one country to another. This practice could worsen the allergy sufferers' state of health, especially if they are asthmatic. The countries where they regularly disinfect passenger aircraft cabins are in Latin America, the Caribbean, Australia, and the South Pacific regions. To obtain more information about sanitizing methods in planes, contact your travel agent or the airline company concerned.

On board

• Before beginning a long journey by ship or cruise liner, it is best to find out what kind of medical staff are aboard.

• If the allergy sufferer has skin inflammations, it is important to know that exposure to water can exacerbate the symptoms. To remedy this, you should ask the doctor to prescribe the appropriate protective skin creams.

In the mountains

• People with asthma should be very careful when choosing alpine sports, especially if they are strenuous.

• When going climbing, asthma sufferers should be aware that, above about 15,000 feet (4,500 m) in altitude, the oxygen level in the air is reduced, which is why it may be necessary to bring additional oxygen.

Ask how your meals have been prepared, since food often contains concealed ingredients such as peanuts, eggs, milk, and shellfish that can provoke severe and very serious allergic reactions.

• When practicing winter sports, like skiing, asthmatics should be aware that cold air can irritate their airways and trigger asthma attacks.

• It is advisable to bring with you in your backpack all the medications necessary in case of an allergic attack.

When camping

Among the dangers in camping areas are pollen and insect stings, especially bees and wasps.

• People allergic to pollen should avoid going to the countryside during the pollen season.

• Allergy sufferers should also bring with them the medication to use in case of an allergic reaction; this is especially important for people who are sensitive to insect stings, since this type of medication should be taken immediately after the sting, to avoid more serious symptoms.

Allergies during the Christmas season

• At Christmas, the climate is at its coldest, which causes rooms to be closed and poorly ventilated, with dust mites in the Christmas decorations and the dry decorative flowers, mold on Christmas trees and firewood, and irritation that can be caused by the fragrances of aromatic candles.

• It is advisable to avoid these types of decorations or remove them when the allergy sufferer is not present, wash them with soap and water, if possible, and then put them back.

• If you are allergic to the far and dandruff of animals, it is best to avoid visiting a house with pets, otherwise your enjoyment of the festivities could be spoiled.

Other considerations

• Allergy sufferers should carry the telephone number of their doctor with them.

• Museums tend to have higher than normal concentrations of dust mites, so it is best to visit them as little as possible during the trip.

• Bus terminals and some city areas, such as certain large squares and avenues, often have very high levels of contamination and so you should avoid them, or spend as little time there as possible.

• Allergy sufferers are advised not to spend their vacations in places where they are going to be in direct contact with animals, such as dogs, cats, chickens, and horses, etc. If this is unavoidable, the animals should be prevented from entering the house where the allergic person is staying and especially from entering the sufferer's room.

• People allergic to certain foods should avoid consuming such things as coffee, hot or very spicy food, as well as shellfish, tomato sauces, eggs and their derivatives, spiced processed meats, and alcohol.

• You should avoid, or remain for as little time as possible in very cold rooms, or air-conditioned rooms in very hot weather, since these atmospheres can irritate your airways.

• Before traveling, ask your doctor about the medication you will need during your trip; he will advise you whether you should continue with the same doses or if it is better to change them.

• It is advisable to take out international medical insurance when you are going to travel abroad.

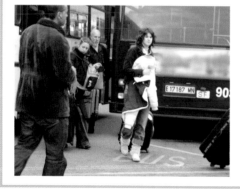

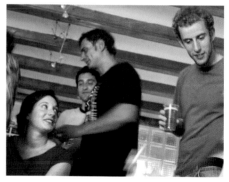

Choking and asphyxia

Obstruction to the airways by foreign bodies, whether in the form of food or otherwise, can cause asphyxia, since this prevents oxygen contained in the air from reaching the lungs. If the problem is not dealt with swiftly, the brain will not receive sufficient oxygen, leading to loss of consciousness and even to death.

Choking and asphyxia

Choking accidents can endanger life, since obstruction of the airways (whether of the throat, trachea, or bronchial tubes) causes asphyxia and loss of consciousness.

Asphyxia through obstruction of the airways is caused by the inhalation of solid bodies, such as badly chewed food, small toys, buttons, coins, dentures, and even vomit, which interrupts the normal breathing process and may even lead to death.

These accidents happen suddenly and usually require urgent assistance.

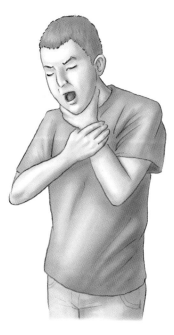

The universal choking reflex

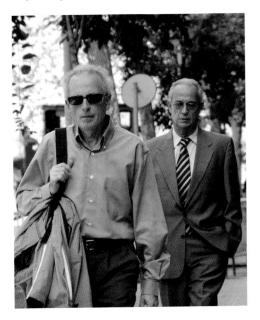

The obstruction can be of two types, incomplete or complete, and affects both conscious and unconscious people.

Partial obstruction

• When the obstruction is partial or incomplete, the victim can continue breathing and inhale a sufficient quantity of air to be able to cough. If the person is able to cough energetically, there is no reason to be alarmed. The coughing mechanism will cause the foreign body to be expelled.

167

The Heimlich maneuver

Some years ago, a technique was developed, called the "Heimlich maneuver," named after the doctor who originated it, whose function is to help expel any foreign body that has lodged in the airways.

It consists of pressing with your fists several times in a rapid manner upon the center of the abdomen, below the ribs. This causes the diaphragm to be displaced upwards, producing increased pressure in the chest and driving out the air that is contained in the lungs, thus removing the foreign body from the airways.

This technique, which has saved many lives, is performed in different ways according to whether the victim is a baby or an adult.

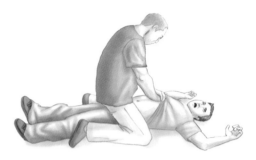

• In the event of partial obstruction, but where the victim can hardly cough or speak and is breathing with difficulty, you must carry out first aid procedures.
• During this type of accident, the victim suffers from pain in the throat and coughing fits, noisy breathing, and difficulty in speaking.

What to do in the case of partial obstruction
• If the victim is conscious and able to cough, it is best to let him carry out the coughing reflex, which in the majority of cases will expel the foreign body.

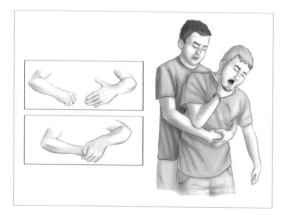

• Do not thump the victim on the back, since this can cause the foreign body to penetrate even further into the airways, leading to total obstruction of the airways.

Complete obstruction
• In the case of total obstruction, the foreign body does not permit air to enter or leave the lungs, so that the person cannot speak, cough, or breathe.
• The individual turns pale in the beginning, then goes a bluish color due to lack of air, raises his hands to his neck—a universal choking reflex—and after about a minute, loses consciousness.
• Other symptoms of choking are swelling in the veins of the face and neck.

What to do in the case of choking
1. When the victim is unconscious or a very obese person:
• If the Heimlich maneuver has not succeeded in expelling the foreign body and the individual has lost consciousness, you must carry out the following procedure:
– Lay the individual on the floor flat on his back with his mouth open.
– Kneel over the individual, at the level of his hips.
– Place one hand with clenched fist two finger-widths above the navel and below the sternum.
– Place the other hand over your first hand, holding the wrist.
– Press sharply and abruptly upwards, in the direction of the lungs, and repeat this 6–8 times.
– Check the victim's mouth to see if the foreign body has been expelled.
– If it has not been expelled, begin cardiopulmonary resuscitation procedures.

2. When the victim is conscious and is an adult:
- Position yourself behind his back and put your arms around his waist.
- Close your right fist and place it over the victim's stomach between the navel and the sternum.
- With your left hand, grasp your right fist.
- Press strongly and abruptly inwards and in the direction of the lungs.
- Release the pressure and repeat the procedure until the victim expels the foreign body.
- In the meantime, ask someone to call the emergency medical services.

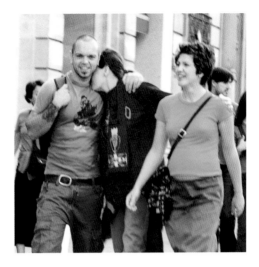

3. When the victim is less than one year old:
- If the baby is able to breathe and cough vigorously:
  - Let him cough, in the hope that the coughing reflex will cure the choking.
  - Stimulate him verbally to make him cough, since this is the most efficient method of expelling any foreign body from the airways.
  - Meanwhile, call the emergency medical services in case they are needed.
  - It is better not to try to extract the foreign body from the baby's airways, since this can have the opposite effect to what you desire and drive the foreign body even further down the airways, thus causing them to be completely obstructed.
  - If the baby has not expelled the foreign body and has stopped coughing, take him urgently to the emergency room, moving him with care.
- If the victim is less than one year old, proceed in the following manner:

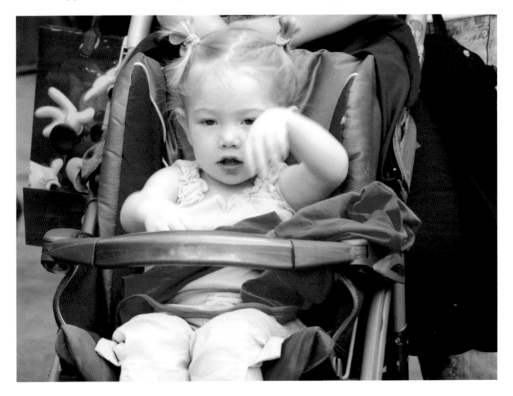

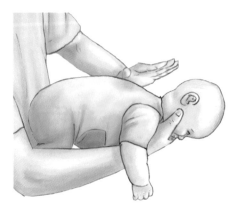

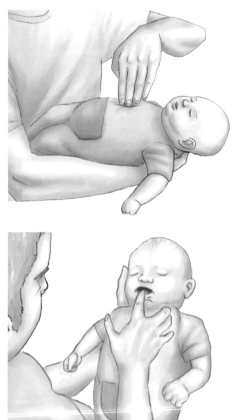

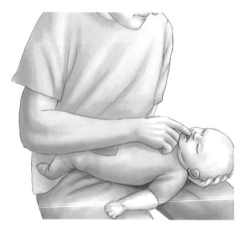

– Above all, keep calm.

– Place the baby on your forearm with his face downwards and his head lower than his trunk.

– Rest his head and shoulders on your right hand.

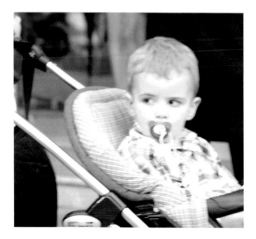

– With your left hand, give him four or five very hard slaps on the back, between the shoulder blades, with the palm of your hand.

– Check if the baby has expelled the foreign body by looking into his mouth.

• If this procedure is unsuccessful, try the following:

– Turn the baby over and hold him on his back.

– Try to keep his head lower than his trunk and looking to one side.

– Place two fingers over his sternum and give him four or five blows pointing upwards in the direction of the lungs so that the air goes up through the trachea and unblocks the airways.

– Check if the baby has expelled the foreign body.

– If the procedure has been unsuccessful, repeat it again.

How to prevent choking and asphyxia

• Chew your food slowly.

• Check the kind of toys that your child plays

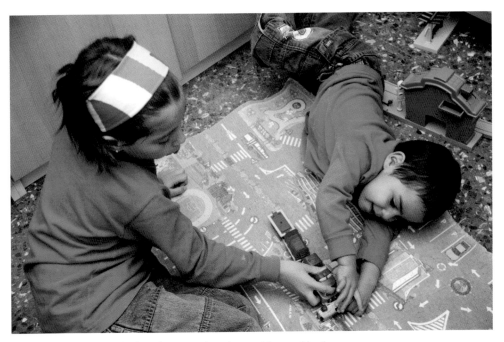

Do not allow children to swim alone; there must always be an adult supervising them.

with, keeping him away from any toys that can be taken to pieces, put into his mouth, and easily choked on.

• Do not allow children to play with plastic bags.

• Do not use cots with bars that a baby can get his head between; the maximum distance between bars should be 2.5 inches (6 cm).

• When putting your baby in a cot, make sure the child has loose clothing on that will not constrict him while he is asleep.

• Babies should sleep on their backs, on a firm flat cot mattress in cots that fulfill the safety norms.

• Do not put necklaces or articles of clothing around the baby's neck.

• Children and adults should not sleep in the same bed.

• Do not leave objects, such as ties, cords, belts, etc. within reach of children in case they wrap them around their necks.

• Make sure you keep your curtain ties tidied away.

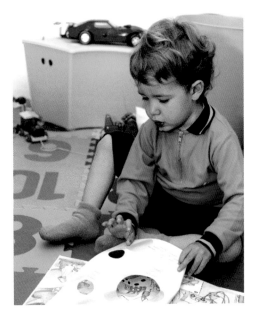

When buying a toy for your child, you should first read the instructions and find out the age for which the toy is recommended. Check that the toy does not have small parts that can fall off and that it complies with international safety regulations.

171

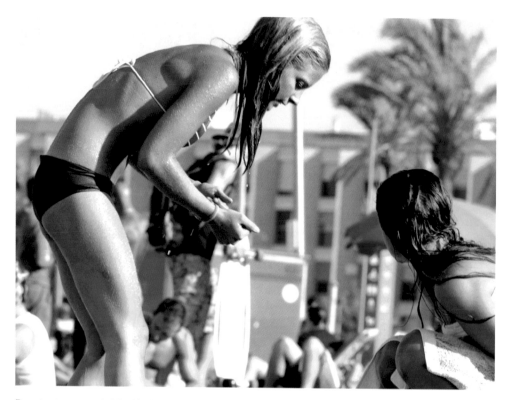

Do not put your trust in inflatable rings or toys, since they can capsize or deflate at an unexpected moment.

• Keep telephone cables rolled up and put away, out of sight of children.

• Never let a child have his bottle alone.

• Supervise your child closely while he is eating.

• Use pacifiers without a string attached. If the pacifier has a string or ribbon, this must be short and should be firmly fixed to the baby's clothing.

• Chopped up food should not be given to children under 3 years old.

• Do not give hard foods or crunchy snacks like peanuts to children less than 3 years old.

• Do not let children run about with objects such as pencils or lollipops in their mouths.

• Do not give babies little things to play with, like coins, buttons, and batteries. Always keep these objects out of reach.

• Teach your children to be polite and well behaved when bathing at the beach or the swimming pool. Teach them not to push other children into the water, not to swim alone, and not to swim in rough weather.

• Private pools must fulfill certain specific safety regulations regarding children. They should be surrounded by a fence that children cannot climb over.

• Always use a baby monitor if you leave a baby sleeping in another room.

Becoming trapped or caught in machinery

Becoming trapped or caught in machinery at home is a very common accident due to our continual contact with equipment that has moving parts or holes into which you can put your fingers. Automatic doors, like those of garages, can also trap people's fingers, especially those of small children who are unaware of the danger.

Becoming trapped or caught in machinery

Closing doors or the moving parts of household appliances often trap fingers. Other more dangerous accidents are caused by parents who are in the habit of sleeping with their children.

Young babies have heads wider than their chests, which is why gaps of between 4 and 8 inches (10 and 20 cm) can be very dangerous, and the baby can get his head stuck and be unable to free himself.

How to prevent children and adults becoming trapped or caught in doors or machinery

• If your child is near a door, window, or balcony with a grille, watch his movements carefully and prevent him putting his fingers where they are hinged or in locking devices.

• When going up or down in an elevator with children, they should be kept back away from the doors.

• If you are going to repair a domestic appliance that could trap fingers, such as a juicer or blender, unplug the apparatus first to prevent it starting up while you are repairing it.

What to do in the case of becoming trapped or caught in machinery

• Disconnect the device in which the person is caught, whether a blender, juicer, or other

machinery. If she cannot get her finger out easily, call the emergency services so that they can extract it in the most suitable manner without causing injury.

• Apply ice to the area to reduce inflammation and speed up the healing process of the injury. The ice should be applied wrapped in a cloth and not put directly on the skin. The ice pack should be kept on the skin for approximately fifteen minutes.

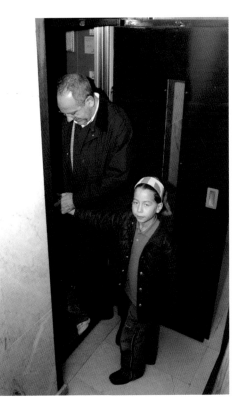

Remind children that the use of elevators by under-age children is absolutely forbidden and that the elevator must only be used in the company of an adult.

Be careful with garage doors

- Automatic garage doors are very dangerous, since they can trap you when opening or closing, or hit people who are near them.

- Garage doors are normally the heaviest item in the home, which brings associated risks, especially for the youngest members of the household, who are not aware of the dangers of the moving parts.

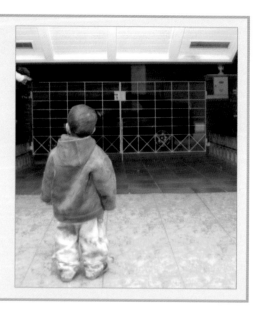

- To avoid the blood remaining trapped in the area of the injury, raise the bruised part above the level of the heart. Thus, if the bruise is on the arm, keep it raised to shoulder level.
- Try to move the affected area as little as possible and not to put it under stress. In the case of children, do not let them run about or do activities that make them use the injured part of the body.
- Do not touch the injury and in the case of bruising, do not drain the blood with needles or similar instruments.

How to avoid becoming trapped in garage doors

- It is very important to teach children that these types of doors are very dangerous. Under no circumstances should children remain near them, especially when they are opening or closing. Parents should keep a safe distance when the doors are opening or closing.
- When the garage door is completely open, children should not be allowed to play under it, due to the danger of it falling on them.
- Children should be taught to ask for an adult's help. When they are old enough, they can be shown how the emergency stop of the garage door works.
- In order to avoid misuse by the youngest children in the household, the controls of the door should be located as high as possible, at least 5 feet (1.5 m) above the ground.

The most typical accidents relating to garage doors involve people's hands or fingers becoming trapped when the garage door is closing.

- Some garage doors have a safety mechanism that makes them open automatically when they encounter an obstacle while closing. It is a good idea to find out if it is possible to install this safety device that is so useful in preventing accidents.

Sleeping with very small children

- Sharing their parents' bed is extremely dangerous for young children, due to the risk of being trapped or crushed under their parents. A child may also be crushed between the mattress and the wall, which can cause severe cases of asphyxiation. For this reason, babies should sleep in their own cot from birth.

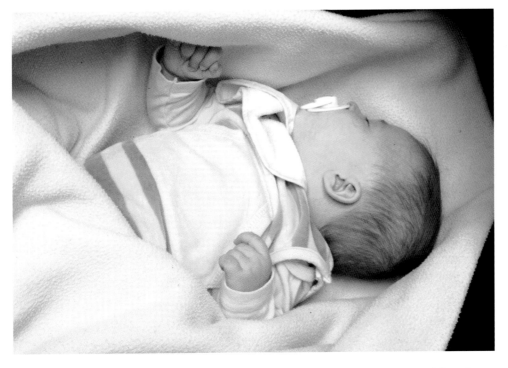

Children should have their own cot from birth and when they are older, they should have a bed the correct size for them.

• All the parts of the garage door, such as the wheels, pulleys, and cables, should be checked regularly. You should not carry out the maintenance yourself; this is much better handled by qualified technicians who, as well as being more experienced, can advise you about the best way of keeping the door in good condition.

How to prevent accidents to children in bed

• To facilitate the mother's breastfeeding and avoid the need to move from room to room that can lead to a mother and child sharing the same bed, it is advisable to put a cot for the baby next to the parents' bed.

• If, despite this advice, a mother decides to sleep with her baby, she should take a series of safety precautions. The baby should not sleep on his stomach, since that position carries a greater risk of the child being crushed. Also, you should not use a mattress that is too soft; it is best if it is as hard as possible. Do not leave bed clothing loose around the bed, to avoid strangulation by the sheets. Position the bed as far away as possible from the wall to prevent the baby becoming caught in the gap.

• Parents who decide to sleep with their children should be aware that they must not take any substances that might put them into a deep sleep.

Travel sickness

Travel sickness due to the motion of various forms of transport, such as cars, ships, or trains, is known as "cinethosis." It is caused by the effect of movement on the inner ear. This form of sickness is very common when traveling and recovery is swift. Each individual has a different susceptibility to travel sickness and this can be aggravated by other factors, such as anxiety.

Travel sickness

Journeys by sea, air, car, or train, often lead to ailments, such as nausea, vomiting, or loss of balance. These symptoms are caused by repetitive acceleration and deceleration. The condition is usually temporary and recovery is swift. This kind of sickness due to movement is more common in small children.

Cinethosis is caused by the sensitivity of the inner ear ducts, called "semicircular canals," which are full of liquid and whose function is to help maintain the body's balance. The sensitivity of the semicircular ducts is hereditary and thus, if parents are prone to suffer from travel sickness, their children probably will as well.

Repetitive and irregular movements cause changes in the liquids inside the semicircular ducts, which send signals of nausea and vomiting to the brain.

Travel sickness is not related to the means of transport used, although it tends to be particularly severe on journeys by car, ship, and airplane.

Factors that may trigger travel sickness:
• The movement of the horizon.
• The poor ventilation of the means of transport, as well as the fumes expelled from the engine.
• Fear, anxiety, and stress.
• Consumption of alcohol.
• Illnesses affecting the ear.

Symptoms of cinethosis:
• Nausea and vomiting.
• Lack of appetite, poor appetite, or no interest in food at all.
• Loss of balance.
• Paleness and an unhealthy complexion.

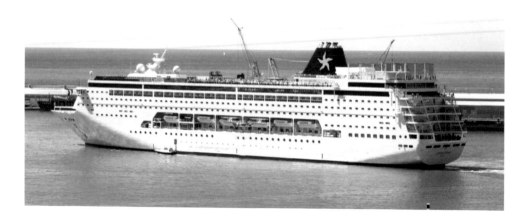

For some people prone to sea sickness, it is helpful to look at the waves when on board.

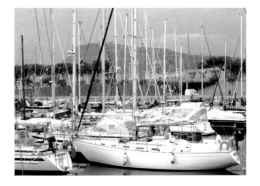

- Yawning.
- Fatigue.
- Cold sweats.
- Accelerated pulse and frequency of breathing.

What should be done in the case of travel sickness?

- When the symptoms begin, breathe strongly and deeply.
- To treat nausea, the best remedy is to lie down, near an appropriate receptacle in case you want to vomit.
- It is also advisable to take a little water in small sips to relieve the stomach symptoms, if you have vomited.
- Generally, you do not vomit more than once and after about four hours, the symptoms tend to disappear.
- To prevent nausea, you can go to the drugstore for anti-nausea medications, which are sold without prescription and are very effective.

General advice for preventing travel sickness

- As a general rule, people who are prone to travel sickness should try to find somewhere on the ship, airplane, or train where they have as little perception of its movement as possible.
- Reading during the journey is not recommended in any situation.
- When traveling, it is best to take up a supine position, that is to say, lying flat on your back with your head well supported. If this position is not possible, try to recline the seat as much as you can.
- Avoid tobacco smoke and smoking areas.
- To improve ventilation, turn on the air-conditioning.
- When traveling by car, try to make the individual who is sick sit in the front seat and look at a fixed point on the horizon. If it is a child, do not let him concentrate on games during car journeys.
- If you are prone to seasickness, it is better to avoid journeys by ship. When this cannot be

avoided, the best solution is to remain on the ship's deck and look at a fixed point on the horizon. Ask for a well-ventilated cabin if you need to sleep.

- When traveling by plane, it is best to ask for a seat near the wings, because in that area of the plane, you are less aware of movement.
- If a child is prone to sickness and visits an amusement park, he should avoid merry-go-rounds and other attractions that make circular movements.
- Your diet before or on a journey should consist of light food with little bulk. Heavy meals increase the risk of sickness. Take liquids to avoid dehydration, but always in little sips, because swallowing large amounts could cause abdominal distension that leads to vomiting. Do not drink alcohol, either. When traveling by plane, avoid sodas.

Overcoming the fear of flying

- One in every six passengers experiences fear, anxiety, and claustrophobia when getting onto a plane. In some cases, it is necessary to seek the help of a specialist to overcome this fear, which is known as "aerophobia." However, by practicing certain relaxation techniques, this phobia can usually be overcome.
- In the majority of cases, fear of flying hides other deeper anxieties, which are externalized in the form of the fear associated with flying.

Travelers with fear of flying explain that, when getting on board a plane, they remember aircraft accidents they have seen on television, they have a sense of danger at being so high, any little noise or problem worries them, or they have no confidence in the pilot.

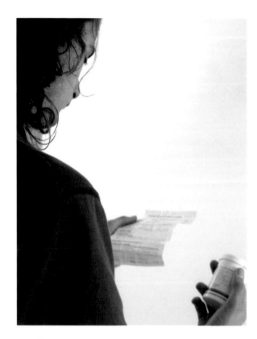

When you are going to drive and are prone to travel sickness, read the instructions of the travel sickness medications, since some of them induce drowsiness and are thus contraindicated.

– During take off and landing, make conversation with the passenger next to you.

– If you are nervous, share your fears with the cabin crew; they are accustomed to this type of situation and know how to give you appropriate assistance.

– If possible, travel in the company of someone you trust.

– Have confidence in the pilots, since they are highly qualified professionals both mentally and physically.

– Remember that, according to statistics, air travel is the safest means of transport there is.

– Do not take stimulants before the flight and ask for an aisle seat.

• There are a series of rules that you can follow to help dispel all the anxiety associated with the fear of flying and transform a plane journey into a genuinely pleasurable experience:

– Breathe strongly and deeply and do not look out of the plane window.

Concentrating on breathing with your abdomen, and doing relaxation exercises with your feet, thighs, hands, arms, neck, and head can help to reduce nervousness when flying.

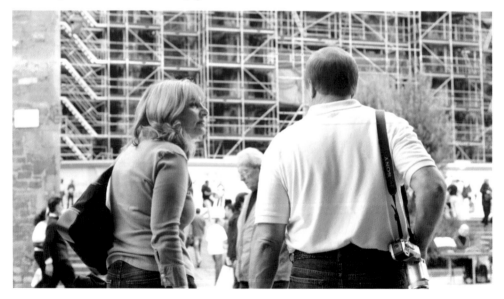

How to avoid accidents and injuries on vacation

Muscular injuries and fractures on vacation, especially in the mountains, carry more risk than at home, due to the impossibility of taking the victim immediately to the emergency room. For this reason, it is advisable to take every precaution to avoid accidents. If unfortunately one does occur, it is necessary to rely on improvisation and imagination to ensure that the casualty remains in the most favorable state possible until the arrival of the emergency medical services.

Advice for avoiding muscular injuries and fractures on excursions to the beach or the mountains

• Bruises are injuries to the muscular tissue that cause pain, inflammation, and a dark or purple color in the skin.

• Sprains and twisting injuries involve the stretching of the ligaments around the joints and if the sprain has been severe, the ligaments may break completely or partially. The symptoms are pain and inflammation.

• If the pain and swelling continue, the victim should be taken to the emergency medical services, so that they can assess the state of the injury and provide suitable treatment.

• A fracture can be simple or compound—in the latter case, the bone breaks through the skin. Broken bones may remain aligned or may get out of alignment with each other, due to the tensions that the surrounding muscles are subjected to.

• Bone fractures tend to be very painful, producing inflammation and a purple coloration of the skin. In the case of fractures, there should be no movement in the injured area to avoid aggravating the situation and the casualty should be taken immediately to the emergency medical

services for assessment and appropriate treatment.

• It is generally difficult to avoid this type of injury during vacations on the beach or in the mountains, but you can follow certain recommended steps to avoid accidents.

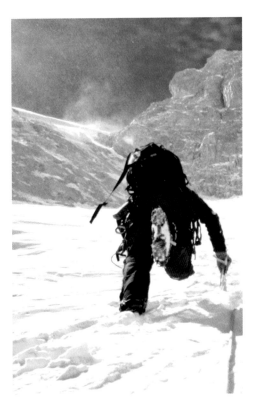

If an accident happens in the mountains, mark out the site well so that you can locate the victim when you return.

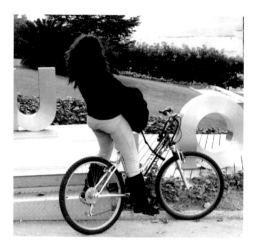

All divers should display a buoy on the surface indicating their presence; this is very important to avoid collisions with motor launches and boats.

• Never leave the injured person alone. If this is unavoidable, because you have to go for help, leave the victim well covered up and with a supply of food and drink.

What to do in the case of an accident in the mountains

• Remain calm, do not spread fear to the others around you, or to the victim.

• Carry out the first aid techniques suitable for the type of injury concerned.

Alert the emergency or civil rescue services. For this purpose, it is useful to take a cell phone on trips. If there is no cell phone available, ask one person to go to the nearest refuge or village in search of help.

Avoiding accidents when participating in adventure sports

How to avoid accidents when climbing

• Rock climbing carries the risk of very serious falls, which is why safety methods are used to ensure that when this happens, the climber does not go into an uncontrolled fall.

• Climbing requires a very comprehensive knowledge of its techniques, so it is not advisable to engage in this sport unless you are

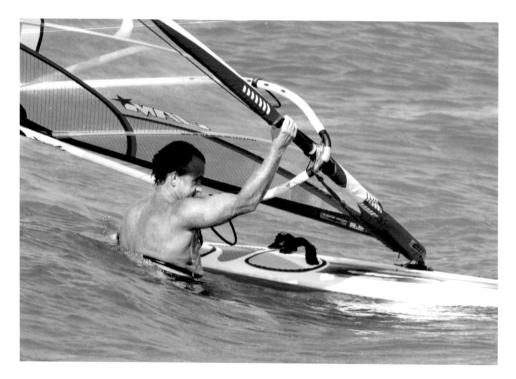

What information should be given when calling the mountain emergency services

- A description of the accident, the number of victims, the type of injuries sustained and their apparent severity.
- The place and time when the accident occurred. If you do not know the exact spot, you can give reference points: whether it is near a river, beside a cliff, or in a forest clearing, etc.
- The full names of the victims, whether they are experienced hikers and what they are wearing, etc.

Muscular injuries and bruises improve when ice is applied and the joint is allowed to rest, bandaged up if necessary.

accompanied by an instructor or experienced climber.

- Children and adolescents should always be in the company of adults when climbing.
- Before taking up this sport, you should have knowledge of meteorology.
- Before going climbing, you should undergo a training schedule that develops the necessary muscles. It is not advisable to practice climbing in a vacation area without being fully fit physically, due to the risk of slips and falls.

Preventing accidents when diving

- Before going scuba diving, you should attend a diving course that grants diving licenses, which require knowledge of first aid techniques to carry out in case of accident.

- Ask to see the instructor's qualifications, as well as the diving center's license.
- Ask for new equipment if that is possible and if not, at least make sure that it has had the appropriate regular checks.
- It is prohibited to go diving alone; you must always be in the company of another diver.
- Each certificate sets a limit on the depth to which you are permitted to dive. It is not advisable not to exceed this limit.

How to immobilize fractured limbs

- Immobilize fractures by means of splints.
- While medical assistance is on its way, you can improvise with materials that immobilize the fractured limb. Use pieces of wood, cardboard, newspapers, or metal rods, etc.
- Once the fracture has been put in a splint, the limb should be raised up.
- A joint should be immobilized above and below the injury.

What to do in the case of muscular injuries and bruises

- First, try to reduce the pain. Apply an ice pack (never ice directly) on the affected area for about 15 minutes.
- Try to keep the injured area immobilized.
- If there is a wound, wash it with running water and do not apply creams or ointments.
- If there are no wounds, you can apply an anti-inflammatory and analgesic ointment.

- If the bruising is serious and has occurred on the leg, this should be kept elevated for some hours.
- Do not massage the affected area vigorously or rub it.
- Do not drain the bruises or squeeze them.
- Acetaminophen (Tylenol) or ibuprofen may be taken for the pain, but aspirins are not recommended, since they can increase the size of the bruises.
- If the pain continues and you cannot move the injured body part, go to a medical center.

• If no such material is available, in the case of a broken arm, the fractured limb should be secured to the individual's trunk and with a broken leg, it should be immobilized by securing it to the healthy leg.

• When the fracture has been immobilized, the victim should not be moved from the scene of the accident and should be allowed to rest.

Examples of improvised splints in the mountains

Traumatic mechanisms

• **Direct.** When a certain mechanical element impacts upon part of the body.

• **Indirect.** For example, in a forced movement, such as in the shoulder when a person is left

What to do in the case of a fracture

Normally, fractures recover quickly and easily. It is very important in a fracture to immobilize the injury and follow certain recommended steps to aid full recovery:

• Soothe the pain by applying ice packs.

• Keep the victim in the most comfortable position for him, but avoiding the least movement.

• Do not try to put the broken bone back in place.

• Loosen his clothing, but do not try to remove anything. This should only be done by trained personnel.

• Take the person to the nearest emergency room. If you judge it appropriate, call an ambulance, or transport him yourself supporting the injured limb with a splint.

   If the fracture is compound, wash it with running water if possible and cover it with sterile gauze.

• Do not poke the wound.

• Ask the person if he is vaccinated against tetanus in order to prevent infection.

Splints for the upper limbs

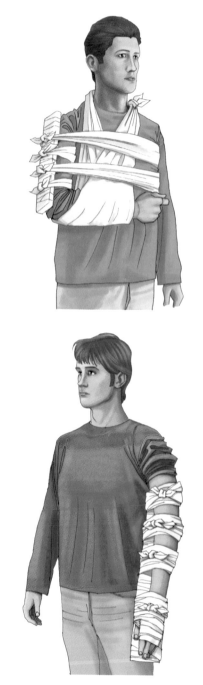

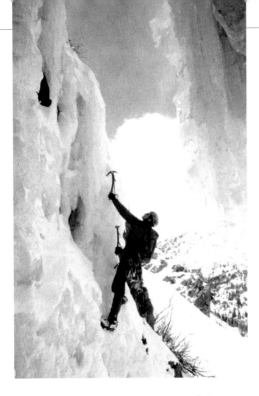

If you envisage hiking or skiing in the mountains at above 6,500 feet (2,000 m) in altitude, consult your doctor about altitude sickness.

— Going into the mountains with defective equipment that does not provide suitable protection from the cold.

— If there has been a fall, which has caused the victim to become immobilized.

— Certain mountain accidents, such as avalanches, etc.

— If the victim has injuries or wounds that do not allow his body to regulate his temperature.

— The speed at which the body temperature falls; if this has been sudden, the hypothermia is more severe.

— If the victim's clothing is wet and the wind is very strong, this accelerates the process of hypothermia.

— If the individual remains submerged in cold water.

What should be done in the case of hypothermia?

• Insulate the victim from the ground, either with thermal blankets or insulating sheets.

• If an aluminum or survival blanket is available, place this over the victim. The function of these blankets is to reflect the heat emitted by the individual.

• If his clothing is wet, remove them and change them for dry clothes.

• Whoever is helping should hug the victim to transmit their body heat to him.

• Hot water bottles can be prepared and applied to the victim, always making sure that the temperature is not extreme and does not cause burns.

• Do not move the victim and if you must, do it very gently, since the heart, in cases of hypothermia, cannot tolerate strain; this can even cause cardiac arrest.

• If the victim is still conscious, give him warm or very sweet liquids.

• Call the emergency medical services to collect the victim.

Altitude sickness

• Climbing to the summits of mountains is a very risky challenge, which can adversely affect your health. As you ascend, the oxygen become scarcer and causes so-called "altitude sickness," a condition that occurs because the body is not yet adapted to the lack of oxygen. This is more frequent in people who do not normally live at above 6,500 feet (2,000 m). If an individual remains at a very high altitude for a long time, his body becomes accustomed to the low levels of oxygen and this condition disappears.

• A quarter of individuals who go above 6,500 feet (2,000 m), and more than half of those who go above 13,000 feet (4,000 m) suffer from altitude sickness.

• Altitude sickness is a condition that occurs quickly, after a few hours of climbing; it normally disappears after two to three days.

• There are other factors, particular to each individual, which cause this condition.

To prevent serious injuries, children should always be suitably protected by a helmet when skiing.

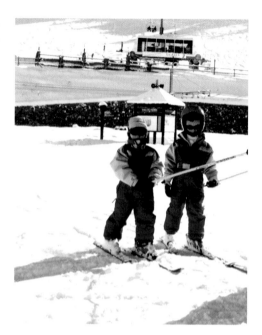

The symptoms of altitude sickness

• When altitude sickness is mild, it causes weakness, headache, nausea and vomiting, fatigue, difficulty in sleeping, and gastrointestinal upsets. These symptoms disappear when the body has adapted to the new altitude.

• When the altitude sickness is more severe, it can cause alterations in the mental state of the person, lack of motor coordination, and inflammation of the legs.

• The symptoms of altitude sickness should not be ignored, since they can develop into a serious condition and even cause death in some cases.

How to prevent altitude sickness

• When traveling at high altitudes, if possible, you should allow your body to adjust, ascending

Before going down a ski run, you should do stretching and warming-up exercises. If not, you may get injured.

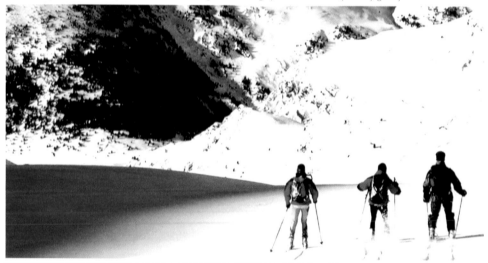

What to do in the case of altitude sickness

• It is best to descend immediately to a lower altitude, but if the symptoms are mild and easily bearable, you can stay at the same altitude and let your body adapt gradually, resting and avoiding exercise.

• If the symptoms are severe, it is advisable to reduce altitude and observe if the symptoms improve. You should carry on descending until the symptoms have disappeared.

• It is not advisable to ascend again until the symptoms have totally disappeared.

• You should also avoid dehydration, which causes fatigue.

Ski injuries

- Skiing carries risks if you fail to take due precautions, such as previous physical preparation and obtaining suitable equipment.
- More than half of injuries caused by skiing occur to the lower limbs, especially the knees; these affect women most. The rest occur in the shoulders, elbows, wrists, head, and spine.

- The most frequent injuries, such as sprains or dislocations, do not tend to be serious, but more serious injuries can also occur, such as ruptured ligaments or cartilages.

gradually. An individual in a good state of health can ascend to 6,500 feet (2,000 m) without any problem. However, when going above 6,500 feet, the best thing is to ascend at a rate of about 1,000 feet (300 m) per day, so that the body can adapt gradually. This is especially recommended if you normally live close to sea level.

What should you do when traveling with children?

- In general, there are no problems traveling with children at high altitudes, but it is quite likely that they will suffer from altitude sickness, since their bodies are smaller and more sensitive to variations in oxygen, making it harder for them to adapt than an adult.
- Parents and adults who accompany children to high places should be especially vigilant regarding the symptoms that may occur and be able to recognize them.

Preventing skiing injuries

- You should warm up your muscles before skiing, making circular movements with your legs and arms for five minutes. It is also helpful to do a little running.
- Take special care at the beginning and end of the ski run, since these are the times when muscles are most prone to injury. At the beginning, because the muscles are cold, and at the end, due to muscular fatigue.
- Take a rest every two hours to allow your muscles to recover.
- Given that during skiing you lose a lot of liquids and mineral salts due to sweating, it is advisable to take isotonic drinks and foods with a high energy content, such as bananas and dried fruit. Alcohol is not recommended and neither are bulky meals.
- You must be very sure of your abilities before going down difficult ski runs; it is advisable not to go too fast.

What to do in case of falls

- Many injuries are caused by the way the skier gets up after a fall, rather than the fall itself.
- After a fall, if you notice an intense pain when

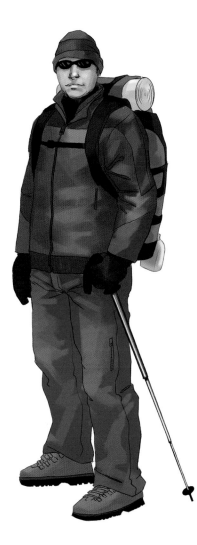

Necessary equipment for the mountains

When hiking in the mountains, you should take the minimum necessary equipment for protection against the sun, wind, and cold, and also an emergency kit. The minimum equipment carried should be the following:

- Backpack. This should be large, suited to your body and with a minimum capacity of 3,500 cubic inches (57 liters approx.). You should try out the backpack in the shop before using it to avoid any future problems.
- Sleeping bag. This should be of good quality and suitable for temperatures of at least as low as 23°F (5°C).
- Insulating sheet. Choose an insulating sheet that protects you against the cold of the ground and that is light, if possible.
- Water bottle. It is advisable to bring 3 pints (1.5 liters) for your personal consumption to avoid dehydration.
- Walking stick. The use of walking sticks is recommended, since they help maintain balance when hiking and make it a more pleasurable, less strenuous activity.
- Footwear. It is important to choose good footwear that does not squeeze your feet and is not too loose. It should also be transpirable (should "breathe") and insulate your feet against the water and cold.
- Gloves. Gloves with a polar lining can be worn. It is advisable to bring a replacement pair in case the others get wet.
- Cap. This should cover your ears and fore-head; a cap with a polar lining is recommended.
- Sunglasses. Buy them from a specialized establishment; they should have higher sun protection than normal sunglasses and very high UV protection.
- High-factor sunscreen. The snow and sun can cause serious burns, as bad as at the beach, or worse.
- Lip protector.
- Flashlight.
- Pants. These should be comfortable, transpirable (should "breathe") and water resistant. Jeans and other cotton pants are not recommended, because they get wet easily.
- T-shirts. These should be comfortable, transpirable and water resistant.
- Jacket. Varieties with a polar lining are recommended, given that their protective and drying-out qualities make them very suitable for the mountains.
- Waterproof jacket and pants.
- Balaclava.
- Neck scarf.
- Socks. These should be bought in a specialized establishment, to avoid the blisters caused by hiking in your ordinary socks.
- First aid kit.
- Cell phone.
- Thermal blanket.
- Candies and dried fruits.
- Mirror for making signals.
- Whistle.
- Waterproof matches.
- Map of the area where you are going.

you try to stand up, stop trying to get up and wait until the rescue team arrives.

- In the meantime, apply cold to the affected area—use some snow.

Preventing eye injuries

- A very common eye injury among skiers is "photophthalmia," which consists of an irritation to the ocular conjunctiva. It appears after four or five hours of unprotected exposure to the sun and causes reddening of the eyes, a gritty sensation in them, and tears.

- Skiers should also protect themselves against the harmful effects of the sun with glasses designed for skiing, with better anti-UVA ray filters than conventional sunglasses.

Other considerations

- Sunburn can become extremely serious. That is why it is very important to put on a high protection sun cream.
- People with insect bite, pollen, and other allergies should take with them the drugs prescribed by the doctor.

First aid on the beach

The beach is a gathering place where many activities bring certain risks. However, the majority of these risks, such as sunburn, can be avoided by taking some minimal precautions. Other risks, such as being stung by marine animals, are beyond our control.

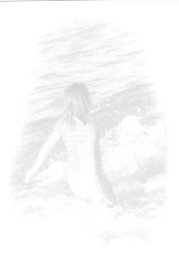

Heatstroke

• You should be particularly aware of the symptoms of heatstroke, since if not treated in time, it can prove fatal.

• Heatstroke or sunstroke results from the failure of your system to produce enough sweat to reduce body temperature, causing it to rise as high as 106°F (41°C) or more.

• If the sweating mechanism stops functioning completely, body temperature can rise to such a point that it may even lead to brain damage and death.

• The capacity to regulate heat is different in each individual. Thus, children have a body refrigeration system that is still undeveloped, and so they are more sensitive to heatstroke. The elderly are also very sensitive.

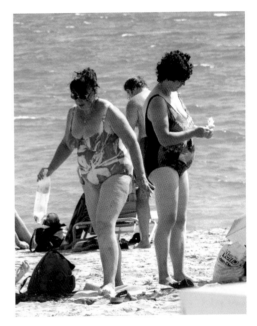

Hydration is very important: you should drink about 4 pints (2 liters) of water a day even if you do not feel like it.

How to prevent heatstroke

• Maintain a good level of hydration, drink about 4 pints (2 liters) of water a day. It is essential to drink even if you do not feel thirsty.

• For clothing, wear thin, light garments, with pale colors if possible.

• At home, keep the rooms well ventilated or use the air-conditioning.

• Do not drink alcohol or drinks that contain caffeine.

• Children older than six months can be taken to the beach, but with high sun protection, factor 20 at least.

• The sunscreen should be applied before leaving the house.

• Your head should be protected from the sun, especially in the case of children.

• During the day, eat a variety of light snacks, instead of one or two heavy meals.

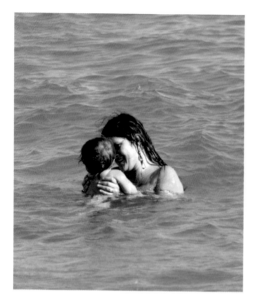

It is not advisable to take babies less than six months old to the beach, since their system of body refrigeration is still undeveloped.

What to do in the event of heatstroke

- The best advice is to prevent it happening altogether.
- Call the emergency medical services to take the victim to hospital.
- Keep the person lying down with his head to one side.
- Remove his clothes. In the meantime, cool his body down, applying wet sheets or cloths over him.
- You can also submerge the person in a bathtub of cold water.
- If ice is available, place ice packs over the wrists and ankles, armpits and neck. In this way, you can cool the main blood vessels. Massage the body while applying the ice so that the blood transfers the cold temperature to the body.

- The symptoms of heatstroke are:

  – The skin becomes red, very hot, and dry.
  – The person's state of consciousness changes, they are irritable and confused.
  – The pulse accelerates and becomes weak.
  – In the case of severe hyperthermia, convulsions may occur.

Dehydration

- Dehydration is a condition in which a person loses more liquid than they can replace. People lose liquid in the form of sweat, urine, feces, and in certain cases, vomiting or diarrhea.

The symptoms of dehydration are:

- Weakness, fatigue, and excessive tiredness.

- Thirst.

- Dry skin.

- Sticky and dry mouth.

- Production of urine reduced or absent.

- Urine of a dark yellow color.

- Sunken eyes.

- Headache.

- Sickness.

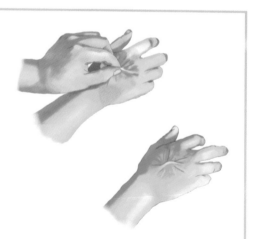

If, when pinching the skin, it remains raised (a condition known as skin turgor), you should go to the emergency room immediately, since this is a sign of advanced dehydration.

Doing intense exercise when the atmospheric temperature and humidity are high can cause heatstroke.

• Babies and the elderly are more prone to suffer dehydration.

• Two-thirds of the body is made up of water and when this quantity falls below the correct levels, dehydration occurs.

How to prevent dehydration

• Drink a least 4 pints (2 liters) of liquid a day, which can be spread between water, milk, and juices, etc.

• Avoid exposure to the sun between 11am and 4pm, since during this period, the rays of the sun are more intense and cause dehydration.

– Eat foods that contain a lot of water, like salads.

– If you feel nausea, stop what you are doing and take a rest for a few minutes with a cool drink.

– If you are going to exercise during the hottest period, you should hydrate yourself before begin-

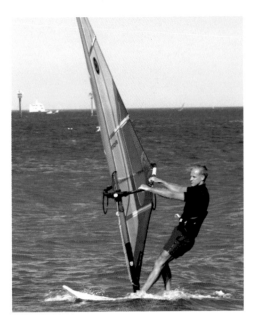

When children go to the beach, to avoid dehydration and heatstroke they should wear light, pale-colored clothing that they can remove easily

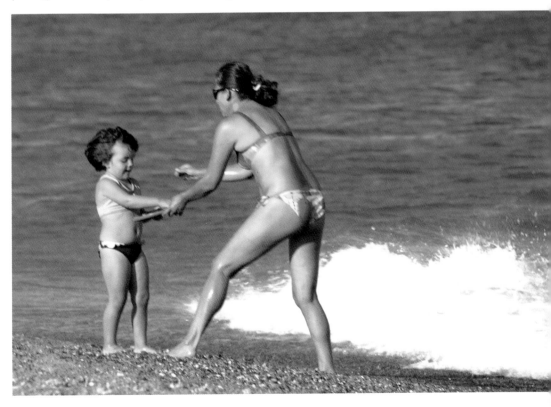

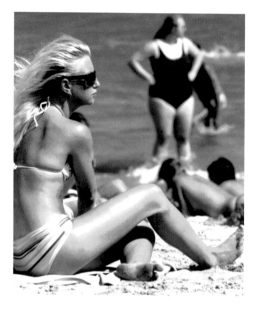

Ultraviolet rays are stronger during the summer months, especially between 11am and 4pm.

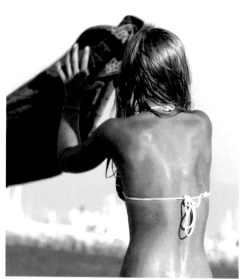

If an individual has sunburn injuries, it is best for him to remain out of the sun until the burns have recovered completely.

ning the activity and continue hydration during the exercise, drinking something cool every 20 minutes approximately.

— Avoid intense exercise during the hottest hours. The best time is first thing in the morning or late in the evening.

Symptoms

The most common symptoms of burns vary between individuals. Below are some of the most usual symptoms:

• The skin becomes red and inflamed.

• Pain and soreness also occur.

• When the burn is more severe, blisters can appear.

• Severe burns can be accompanied by fever, shivering, and weakness.

• Some days after burning, the skin begins to dry up and peel.

What to do in case of dehydration

• The sufferer should immediately stop all physical activity.

• Put the person in a cool, shady place.

• Apply cold water compresses to the body.

• Give them liquid in little sips.

When you should go to the doctor

• In general, dehydration can be remedied by following the home-remedy recommendations given earlier, but there are certain more serious situations that require medical assistance, such as:

• When the person faints each time he tries to get up, even after having drunk liquids.

— In some cases, dehydration can be a sign of more serious problems, like diabetes; trained medical personnel may possibly carry out tests to rule out other illnesses.

Sunburn

• In summer, people expose themselves voluntarily to sunshine with the aim of toning up and bronzing their skin. For this reason, it is important to understand the dangers of the sun.

• Sunlight contains ultraviolet (UV) rays, which damage the skin during excessive exposure to the

Do not forget also to put sunscreen on the places that are often overlooked, such as the ears, lips, the back of the neck, and feet.

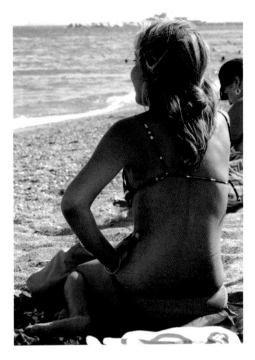

sun. These rays can penetrate the skin causing injuries, which may vary from slight reddening to second-degree burns with blisters.

• In addition to sunburn, ultraviolet rays can cause other long-term problems, such as premature aging of the skin and skin cancer, which is why their effects must be taken seriously.

• People who have very pale skin with frequent moles and freckles and with a family history of cancer, have more chance of developing skin cancer.

• The body has a defense mechanism in the form of melanin skin pigmentation, but when the ultraviolet rays exceed the protective capacity of the pigmentation, burns occur.

• Each individual has a different quantity of melanin. Thus, for example, people with pale skin tolerate the sun less, because they have less melanin.

• Sunburn, unlike thermal burns, does not show symptoms immediately. The pain and reddening usually appear between six and forty-eight hours after sun exposure and peeling begins around three to eight days after exposure.

**What to do
in the case of sunburn**
• If the only symptom is reddening in the area affected, and it covers no more than 10 percent of the body, cold-water compresses can be applied, or highly diluted oxygenated water, or moisturizing cream and corticosteroid creams.

• Consult a pharmacist about using corticosteroid creams to alleviate the inflammation; they will advise on the most suitable type of cream. Do not use the medication unless you are completely sure.

PREVENTING SUNBURN

The best way of preventing sunburn is to protect yourself from the sun's rays. According to the American Academy of Dermatology, you should follow the ABC steps (Avoid, Block, and Cover):

Avoid	Avoid the sun from 11am to 4pm, because this is the time when the sun's rays are most harmful.
Block	Block the sun's rays, using a factor-15 sunblock at least. This should be applied half an hour before going to the beach, and several times throughout the rest of the day. Children less than six months old should not use sunblock.
Cover	Cover yourself from the sun with hats and protective clothing, such as long-sleeved T-shirts. Protect your eyes by wearing sunglasses with high-level solar filtration.

People that get stung by jellyfish become sensitized—if they are stung again, they can experience more severe reactions.

What should you do if you are stung by a jellyfish?

- Do not clean the affected area with freshwater, since this can reactivate the toxin. Use salt water, vinegar, or water mixed with sodium bicarbonate to wash the area.

- Do not rub the area with either sand or a towel.

- Apply cold to the affected area for fifteen minutes, using a plastic bag containing ice. Do not apply the ice directly, since the freshwater from the ice could also reactivate the toxin.

- Analgesics may be taken to alleviate the pain.

- If the injured area does not improve after several ice applications and becomes inflamed, or the victim has fever, go to an emergency room.

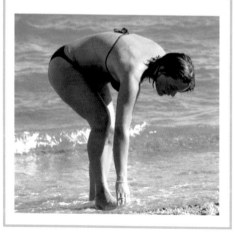

- It is also helpful to submerge yourself in a bathtub of cold water.
- For the pain, analgesics, such as acetaminophen (Tylenol) or aspirin, can be taken.
- Keep the burnt area very clean to avoid infection.
- If blisters appear, do not burst them, since there is a risk they might become infected.
- If the blisters burst, apply an antibacterial ointment over the affected area. Ask the pharmacist to recommend a suitable one in each case.
- If the burn blisters a lot, wash the area well without rubbing, cover it with sterile gauze and go to a medical center.
- Drink lots of water to replace body fluids.

Getting stung by jellyfish and other marine animals
- In summer, sea currents frequently bring jellyfish close to the shore. Getting stung by jellyfish when bathing is therefore a common occurrence.
- When you brush against a jellyfish, it releases a poison that causes reddening of the skin, stinging, and itching.

Sea urchins
- Sea urchins are marine invertebrates with a highly compact shell, formed from very strong calcium plates and covered with spines.
- The only danger from sea urchins is due to the fragility of their spines, which can become embedded in your feet if you step on them.
- If you tread on an urchin, first disinfect the area, after washing it with soap and water.
- Then remove the spines carefully, one by one, with some fine tweezers.
- It is important to extract the spines, since if they remain, it increases the risk of infection.
- If the area becomes infected, go to a medical center, so that specialized staff can remove the spine with suitable instruments.

Bathing precautions

In the summer, it is very common for people to bathe in swimming pools or at beaches that do not conform to minimum health standards. You must be aware of the risks associated with bathing to be able to enjoy vacations by the seaside in complete safety.

Bathing precautions

- Though stomach cramps are easily prevented, they can be extremely serious, which is why they should not be treated lightly.
- Stomach cramps are caused by the lack of blood supply in the digestive system.
- When you have eaten a very heavy meal that is hard to digest, the blood circulation becomes concentrated in the digestive system. If you go abruptly into the water at a beach or pool, while you are digesting, the blood moves suddenly to the rest of the body to counteract the change in temperature produced by the water.
- This condition can also occur when a person is not digesting; for example if the person has been sunbathing for a long time, her skin is burned and she plunges into the water, the difference in temperature between her body and the water can even cause a heart attack.
- The symptoms caused by stomach cramps are varied. Among them are the following:
  - Nausea and vomiting.
  - Fall in blood pressure.
  - Fainting, loss of consciousness.
  - Paleness.

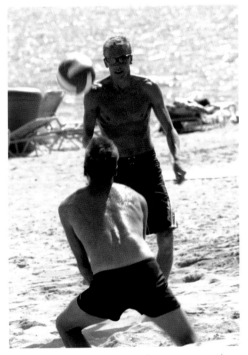

Stomach cramps can also occur during strenuous exercise, while you are digesting your food.

Ice creams and headaches

- Some people get a severe headache from eating ice cream. This happens because you are stimulating a ganglion located at the back of the pallet, which causes a reaction, very similar to a headache. This reaction lasts a couple of minutes at the most and goes away by itself.
- To avoid this unpleasant sensation, you should eat the ice cream slowly and let it melt in your mouth before swallowing.

– Sweating.

– Heart attack in the most severe cases.

In the event of stomach cramps

• Call the emergency medical services immediately.

• If the person is in the water, get them out straight away.

• If the person is unconscious, check their carotid pulse (at the neck—see picture opposite).

If there is no carotid pulse

• If the person has no pulse, begin cardiopulmonary resuscitation procedures.

• Continue this until the emergency medical services arrive.

Preventing stomach cramps

• In the case of stomach cramps, prevention is much easier than cure. By following some simple advice, they can be avoided:

– If you have had a heavy meal, wait about three hours before bathing.

– While you are digesting, do not swim or shower in cold water.

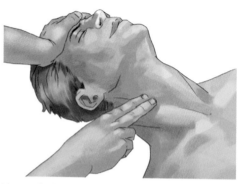
How to check the carotid pulse.

– If you have been sunbathing for a long time, or doing strenuous exercise, do not rush into the water.

– When you go into the water, do it gradually, wetting first your feet and wrists, and then slowly letting your body in, so as to accustom your body to the change in temperature.

– Do not drink very cold drinks in great gulps after strenuous exercise or sunbathing for a long time.

– Get out of the water if you feel nausea or a severe fit of shivering.

Drowning

• Every year, thousands of people die from drowning. Any bather can be affected, whether he is an experienced swimmer or not.

• The term drowning refers to the asphyxia caused by the entry of water into the lungs, which prevents the victim from breathing.

• Statistics reveal that drowning can occur as easily on beaches as in pools and that the principal victims are usually children.

• People can get into a drowning situation for many reasons, the most common being as a result of swimming for long periods of time, which causes muscular fatigue and cramps. Drowning can also occur due to heart and lung failure .

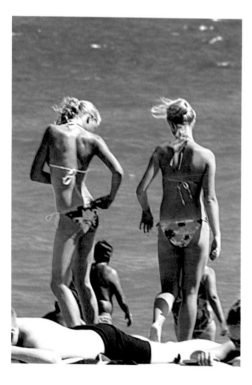

If a child feels a prickling sensation or gets a headache when eating ice cream, advise him not to eat it too fast.

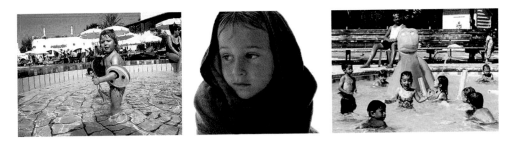

It is advisable to shower before entering the pool to get rid of germs, remains of hair, and protective creams.

What to do
if you see somebody drowning
- Call the lifeguard immediately.
- If the depth of the water allows you to reach the victim, try to make a human chain with the help of other bathers until you can reach the place where the person is in danger.
- When the casualty is back on land, begin cardiopulmonary resuscitation procedures. Before commencing, check that his airways are free of any blockage or object and lean his head backward so as to stop the tongue blocking the throat.
- If you are able to carry out this procedure, you can begin it when you reach a water level where you can stand, with the help of another person. One person supports the head and neck of the victim and the other does mouth-to-mouth resuscitation.

How to prevent drowning
- At the beach, always follow the instructions of the lifeguards.
- Become familiar with the meaning of the warning flags on the beach:

- Do not bathe after very heavy meals.
- Go into the water gradually, not suddenly.
- Do not bathe in very deep water or alone.
- Swim parallel to the shore.
- Watch your children while they are bathing.

Bathing in swimming pools
- Swimming pools can be sources of infections and inflammations if the water treatment is not performed correctly, and there are frequent problems relating to both the lack of and excess of chlorine in the water.
- Nearly half of all the health problems in swimming pools are due to the bad state of the water. For the pool water to remain clean and healthy, it should be free from bacteria and an excess of chlorine. In addition, the acid or alkaline level (the pH level) of the water should be kept within a stable range.
- When bathing in a pool, if you notice stinging in your eyes and a strong smell of chlorine, this means that the pH level of the water is not at permitted levels or that the pool filters are not functioning correctly. To resolve this problem, contact the pool administrator. To alleviate the stinging in

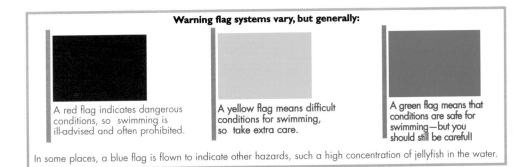

Warning flag systems vary, but generally:

A red flag indicates dangerous conditions, so swimming is ill-advised and often prohibited.

A yellow flag means difficult conditions for swimming, so take extra care.

A green flag means that conditions are safe for swimming—but you should still be careful!

In some places, a blue flag is flown to indicate other hazards, such a high concentration of jellyfish in the water.

your eyes, stop bathing in the pool until the irritation has cleared up.

• Another problem related to exposure to high concentrations of chlorine, is that of dry skin or xerosis, due to the powerful oil-removing effect of the chlorine. The skin looks cracked, fragile, and flaky, especially on the lips, arms, and legs. To remedy this problem, apply moisturizing lotion to the skin after bathing.

Safety advice
for swimming pools

• After eating, wait a reasonable time before getting in the water to avoid stomach cramps and sickness.

• Go into the water gradually without diving, especially after strenuous exercise or prolonged sunbathing.

• Do not bring diving equipment to the pool, such as goggles, flippers, or snorkels, since these can hurt other bathers.

• It is advisable to shower after bathing in the pool to get rid of the remains of chlorine on your skin.

• Always watch children while they are bathing in the pool and do not let them swim alone, even if they are paddling or using a float.

• Do not use inflatable rings that go around the child's waist, since they can easily slipoff. The type of floats that fit on the child's back or inflatable arm bands are preferable.

• Check that anything the child is playing with in the pool is officially approved and accords with the safety regulations.

• Tell your child to dry his ears well after bathing so as to prevent ear infections.

Fungal infections

• Fungal infections are more common in summer, due to the changing of footwear, increased perspiration, and the poor conditions of hygiene at some public swimming pools.

• Damp clothing, synthetic footwear, and walking on unhygienic surfaces, such as sand on the beach, also increases the incidence of fungal infections.

• Fungal infections, also called mycosis, are contagious and if not treated in time can become chron-

The use of abrasive soaps wears away the skin. For your daily shower, use plain soaps with a neutral pH balance.

Care when bathing

Accidents through falling into water constitute another of the important causes of infant mortality and of permanent damaging consequences. These types of accidents generally occur in private or public swimming pools around which infants and small children play without close supervision by an adult. Such accidents are also common in places where water is stored in tanks, bath tubs, laundries, and buckets, etc., the prognosis being more serious when they contain chemical products, like soaps or disinfectants. Adolescents are particularly prone to this type of accident, following the consumption of alcohol or the use of drugs. The following are some measures for reducing accidents:

• Safety around pools. This can be achieved ideally by fences that prevent free access by children without the company of a responsible adult.

• Pool covers. These are a good alternative since they prevent access by children when the pool is not in use.

• Alarms. There are alarms that activate when an object falls or enters the pool.

• Lifesaving training. All those responsible for supervising children in aquatic pursuits should take a course on cardiopulmonary resuscitation for children. This should also be done by anyone who has a pool at their home.

• Special vigilance over children with medical problems. This is essential for those who suffer from convulsive syndromes. They are at very high risk of being involved in accidents, due to the possibility of a crisis occurring while they are in the water.

• When children are playing by pools, lakes, and rivers, etc., they should always be under the supervision of an adult.

ic, since they infiltrate the deeper layers of the skin and become increasingly difficult to get rid of.

• The way mycosis spreads is usually from walking barefoot around the swimming pool and the shower area or through sharing towels.

What are the signs of mycosis

• It usually takes the form of whitish patches that appear on the surface of the skin.

• Other types of fungi cause so-called "athlete's foot," one of the most common and contagious mycotic infections. This fungus causes lesions in the form of peeling skin, bumps, or pinkish areas between the toes and is accompanied by intense itching.

• Another mycotic infection that can be contracted when walking barefoot in areas near the water is "plantar warts" or "veruccas." These are flat warts on the sole of the foot and can be painful when walking.

What to do in the case of fungal infections

Consult your doctor so that he can recommend anti-fungal or anti-mycotic products. The treatment

usually lasts between one and three weeks.

How to avoid fungal infections

• Each time after you have been in contact with the pool water and after each swim, it is advisable to dry your feet very well, especially between your toes and under your nails. The aim is to keep your skin dry all the time.

• Use footwear that allows your feet to "breathe."

• Avoid underwear made from synthetic material. Choose cotton or other natural fabrics. Synthetic fabrics inhibit perspiration.

General advice for hygiene in swimming pools and on the beach

• You should not swim at the beach or pool when you are suffering from any intestinal illness that causes diarrhea, since this can be contagious; this is particularly important in the case of babies.

• Do not swallow water from the sea or pool and do not let water get into your mouth.

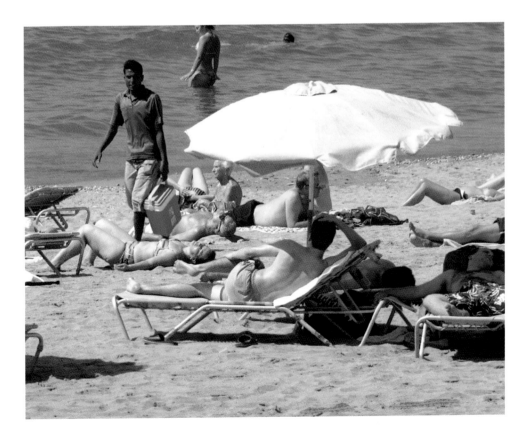

■ Otitis

Otitis from pools or "swimmer's ear" is a very common infection that results from contaminated or excessively chlorinated water. Humidity in the inner ear caused by bathing or showering increases the flakiness of the skin inside the auditory canal, creating a favorable environment for germs to breed. Itching leads to lesions through excessive scratching.

Although it is mainly bacteria that infect the ear, it is very common to find fungi there. Such a condition is often very painful, causing suppuration and inflammation of the auricular chamber and sometimes even affecting hearing. Treatment with antibiotic eardrops is very effective.

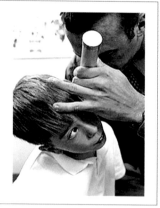

• Do not share towels at the beach or pool.

• Help to keep the beaches and pools clean, using the trashcans and waste containers. Use disposable ashtrays on the beach.

• If you suffer from a contagious disease, it is better not to visit beaches or pools, due to the risk of infecting others.

• In swimming pools, it is not advisable to consume food; do this in the eating areas.

• Do not go through to the pool in your street shoes.

• Do not bring animals to pools, except in the case of guide dogs.

• In the pool, protect your eyes from the chlorine with swimming goggles.

• In the pool, always wear a cap, especially if you have long hair. In sports facilities, this is sometimes obligatory.

• When walking around the pool, wear rubber-soled shoes that prevent slipping and protect you from the wet floor.

Effects of chlorine in swimming pools

Chlorine is a powerful disinfectant used for treating drinking water and pools. It can cause irritation in children with dry skin. This effect can be reduced by a shower in fresh water or a little moisturizing cream applied after bathing.

Acne is also frequent in adolescents exposed for long periods to low concentrations of chlorine.

In children who swim with their eyes open, chlorine can cause chemical conjunctivitis through irritation of the mucus linings. Because it is a bleaching agent, it can bleach your hair if bathing and exposure to the sun are excessive.

Blond people who bathe frequently in pools can get a green tint in their hair.

Accidents during pregnancy

Pregnancy is one of the happiest, and most enriching phases in a woman's life. The vast majority of pregnancies do not present any problem and giving birth is much easier and less traumatic than before, thanks to modern medical and technological advances. Nowadays, you only need to take certain precautions and to be alert to any little difficulties that may occur.

Accidents during pregnancy

• During pregnancy, a woman's body puts on weight, due to the growth of her abdomen. Her vertebral column is subjected to greater load and her center of gravity also changes. These factors lead to a greater risk of falling.

• Generally, falls and knocks to pregnant women do not tend to have severe consequences. However, serious traffic accidents or very violent blows can cause the death of the fetus, even if they do not cause the death of the mother.

• Falls in pregnant women usually occur during the last three months of pregnancy, when the mother is considerably less agile, due to sickness and even sporadic fainting fits. Fainting in pregnant women is caused by changes in blood

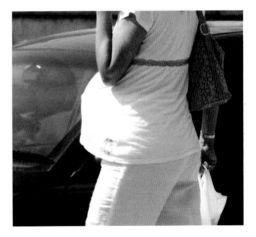

You should wear anything comfortable that is not too tight Using flat shoes or those that have low heels can help to maintain balance and prevent falls.

How can you detect a miscarriage?

The usual symptoms of a miscarriage are:

• Vaginal bleeding.

• Pains in the lower part of the abdomen.

• Loss of sensitivity in the breasts.

• Abrupt disappearance of nausea and morning sickness, if these were present.

• However, this does not mean that the fetus has definitely been lost, because there are cases of some mothers who have discharges of

blood and abdominal pains without any consequences. Nevertheless, if you experience these symptoms, go to the doctor immediately to rule out any possible complications.

• If the mother has nausea and vomiting daily during the first trimester and suddenly stops suffering from this in the second month, there is a possibility that the fetus has been lost, if any of the other relevant symptoms are present. You should go immediately to the doctor so that he can carry out the appropriate tests.

pressure through sudden movements, among other things.

• The fetus is surrounded by amniotic fluid, which acts as a protector and shock absorber against blows. Thus, if the mother receives a light or moderate blow in the abdomen, the amniotic fluid will lessen the impact.

How do you detect premature birth?

• Normally, birth takes place between the 38th and 42nd week of pregnancy. However, on some occasions the moment of birth may come early. For this reason, it is important to know what the symptoms are and call the emergency medical services urgently, given that these types of births tend to be dangerous for the newborn child. As a premature baby, he will need special care.

• Alert the gynecologist immediately if the following symptoms occur:

– Vaginal discharges, which can be in the form of mucus, blood, or watery fluids.

– Frequent uterine contractions.

– Abdominal cramps, which may be accompanied by diarrhea, or not.

– Back pains, especially in the lower back.

– A sensation of pressure in the pelvis.

Emergency births

• The dilation stage of the birth can last many hours. This stage consists of a series of contractions that prepare the opening of the uterus for the baby to emerge. Once the opening of the uterus has dilated completely, you can see the head of the baby in the vagina.

• If it is the mother's first pregnancy, the dilation stage may last sufficiently long for medical assistance to arrive, but for mothers who have had a baby before, this stage can accelerate making the babies head emerge rapidly.

• A sign indicating with great probability that the birth is about to take place is the rupture of the amniotic sac, commonly called "the breaking of the waters." Amniotic fluid looks clear in color and can contain greenish particles. The fluid can come out in small discharges, or all at once.

• Finally, some mothers may have a strong desire to empty their bowels without having felt any pain earlier, which is an unlikely situation. This desire to evacuate comes from the baby's head pressing against the rectum.

Vacations always involve traveling, whether by land, sea or air. Pregnant women are especially advised to avoid long journeys. During the journey, they should stretch their legs, get into a comfortable position and avoid remaining seated for long periods, because they run a greater risk of thrombosis.

It has been demonstrated that smoking during pregnancy causes a reduction in weight of the fetus.

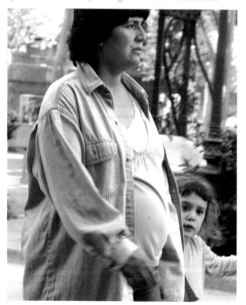

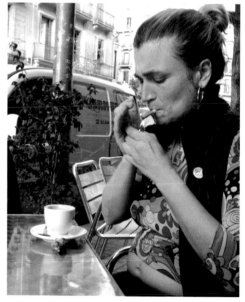

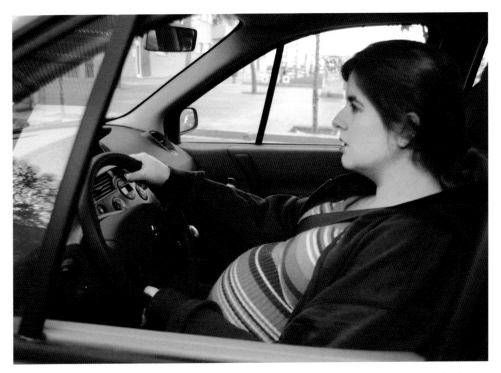

When a pregnant woman travels in a vehicle, she should use a seatbelt. The great majority of car accidents endanger the baby's life. A blow to the abdomen from the steering wheel or a violent fall backward are highly risky for the baby and are even more so if this happens in the last months of pregnancy, since there is a possibility that the placenta will become partially detached from the uterus.

• Call the hospital for medical assistance. If the ambulance does not arrive in time, the mother will have to prepare for an unassisted birth. Fortunately, these types of births are not very common, but it is necessary to know what steps to follow.

What to do
if you are with a woman
when she is giving birth

• Call an ambulance.
• Reassure the mother.
• Advise her to breathe deeply so as to control her impulses to push out the baby. In this way, the baby's birth can be delayed a few minutes, at least until the medical services arrive.
• If after this, the ambulance has still not arrived, the person assisting at the birth should wash their hands, as well as the vaginal area of the mother. Use soap and water.

• If available, wear sterile latex gloves.
• Select a place for the birth. A bed is recommended, or the floor, or any large wide surface. It must be well lit and the temperature should be warm. The place chosen should allow the buttocks of the mother to be slightly raised above the rest of her body.
• Lay out sheets, towels, or clean linen over the site chosen.
• Remove any clothing that might be uncomfortable for the mother.
• Provide her with pillows, cushions, or folded linen to rest her head on and the upper part of her back.
• The mother should lie down with her knees bent.
• At the moment of each contraction, the mother should breathe deeply, exhaling and inhaling strongly, pushing, and counting up to ten.
• She should only push during the contractions, never between them.

How can risks be avoided?

- In general, you should reduce all physical activity and avoid exposure to noxious or contaminating substances.

- If the mother has not had the typical childhood illnesses, such as measles, chickenpox, or rubella, she should avoid contact with people or children who are going through that infectious phase.

- It has been demonstrated that the consumption of alcohol during pregnancy, especially during the first trimester, can lead to congenital malformations.

- From the third trimester onward, due to the abdomen's expansion and a changed center of gravity, you should avoid practicing sports that require balance, such as skiing, skating, and dancing, etc., since these increase the risk of falls.

- If the mother has a profession in which she is exposed to chemical substances, she should consult her specialist regarding precautions she needs to take and the risks involved.

- When the baby's head begins to appear, do not pull on it. Never make any abrupt movements. Tell the mother to stop pushing for a moment, so that you can clean the nose and mouth of the baby, which must be done with a dry towel.
- Support the baby's head with both hands and assist him with a gentle downward movement to help the first shoulder to emerge.
- When the first shoulder is out, gently guide the baby upward, supporting his head while the rest of his body is emerging. It normally comes out by itself.

- Wrap the baby in a clean towel or sheet and place him on the mother's belly.
- Do not stretch the umbilical cord, or cut it. It is also not advisable to separate it from the placenta.
- Keep the mother and baby comfortable in a warm atmosphere until medical assistance arrives.

What to do if you are giving birth and you are on your own
- Call an ambulance.
- Keep calm.

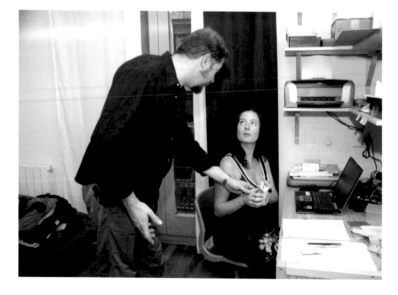

Premature births can occur in women with no previous history and in pregnancies that are progressing normally.

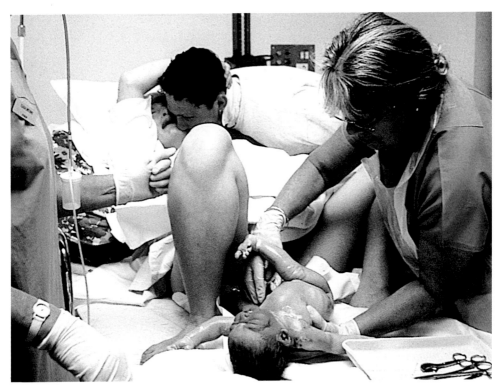

During normal birth, the head of the baby is the first part to come out, followed by the shoulders and the rest of the body. Later, the placenta emerges.

• Practice deep breathing with the aim of controlling your impulse to push out the baby. In this way, the birth may be delayed a few minutes, at least until the medical services arrive.

• Wash your hands with soap and water, as well as your vaginal and anal areas.

• Place clean sheets, towels, or linen over the bed or floor, continuing to breathe deeply all the time, and lie down.

• Wait for medical assistance to arrive while continuing to breathe deeply.

• If you notice that the baby's head is coming out, take advantage of the contractions to help him out, assisting him gently with your hands.

What to do if the woman giving birth is in a car

• If the mother is driving and notices signs of giving birth, she should stop the vehicle immediately and call the emergency medical services.

• She should lie down in the back seat of the car, putting covers or travel blankets under her head and back.

• Observe the procedures described above.

Breathing techniques for controlling the contractions

• Inhale deeply.

• Exhale the air in a gasp or repeated blowing.

What should be avoided during an emergency birth?

• Trying to delay the birth. Do not try to delay the birth in any way at all, by crossing the mother's legs or pushing the baby's head back into the vagina, since this can damage the baby seriously.

• Allowing the mother to go to the toilet. Explain that the feeling of wanting to go to the toilet is a sign that the baby is coming.

• Allowing the mother to push strenuously before you see that the vagina is becoming enlarged with the baby's head. If the mother pushes before the opening of the uterus is completely dilated, this may become torn.

• Pulling the baby out of the vagina. This could seriously injure the mother and baby.

As the probable date of birth approaches, you should begin to think about all the possible situations that may arise when taking the mother-to-be to hospital so as to avoid the possibility of delaying her arrival. Such situations are very rare. There always seems to be time to get to hospital.

• Pulling on the umbilical cord. This forces the placenta to detach, causing severe hemorrhage.

• Cutting the umbilical cord, unless indicated by a doctor.

• Allowing anyone to cough or sneeze over the mother and baby. People with colds, unwashed hands, or open wounds should keep away.

• Using chemical or antiseptic products around the mother or baby. Soap and water are best, since other products may have toxic effects.

What are the symptoms of giving birth?

To identify an emergency birth, the following symptoms should be present:

• Regular contractions. Less than two minutes apart, counted from the start of the first contraction to the beginning of the second.

• A feeling of needing to empty the bowels, caused by the baby's head pressing on the rectum.

• A strong need to push out. The mother realizes that the baby is about to arrive and wants to push it out.

• Bulging vaginal aperture. The baby's head may even be seen during the contractions, as it enters the vagina between each contraction.

• Pushing and effort on the part of the mother. The mother cannot resist the natural instinct to give birth.

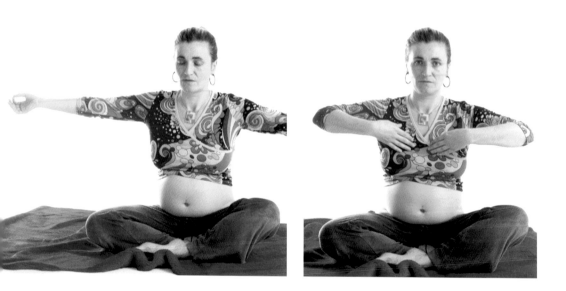

Contraceptive failure

Condoms are used widely to avoid the spread of sexually transmitted diseases, as well as to prevent unwanted pregnancies. Sometimes, however, either as a result of careless behavior during sex, or due to a condom being faulty, it can burst, change position, and even slip off altogether. It is then necessary to use emergency methods of contraception. In these situations, it is best to consult a doctor.

What should you do if the condom bursts or remains inside the vagina?

• Condoms sold to the public are manufactured under strict quality and safety controls, in accordance with health and consumer regulations relevant in each country, thus making it considerably less likely for one of them to burst.

• It is calculated that the probability of a condom bursting is 2 percent.

• If a condom bursts, go immediately to a family planning center to get advice.

• You should visit the family planning center within 72 hours of the incident happening to avoid the risk of an unwanted pregnancy.

• If you do not know a family planning center or there is not one available, ask for an immediate appointment with a gynecologist or an expert doctor.

Why do condoms burst?

• According to statistics, less than 2 percent burst due to faulty manufacture. This is therefore not the most usual cause for a condom to fail.

• In the majority of cases, it happens as a result

of using condoms that are past their expiration date. If coitus is very violent, this can also cause the condom to burst. Another reason is that people often use condoms that are too small.

• The use of unsuitable lubricants can also affect the quality of the condom. You should generally avoid all lubricants based on oily substances: oils and other greasy materials weaken the latex and reduce its resistance by approximately 90 percent. Only those lubricants that are soluble in water are compatible with condoms.

The morning-after pill

• If a condom bursts, it is advisable to take the

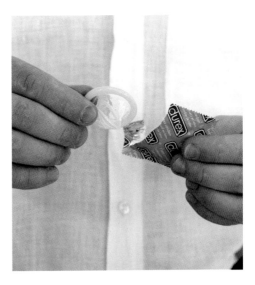

A male contraceptive or condom is a very thin, resistant sheath that is placed on the penis when it is erect. At the moment of ejaculation, the semen collects inside the condom, thus being prevented from penetrating the vagina. The sperm are therefore unable to fertilize the female egg.

How to put on a condom correctly

- Always have condoms available in sufficient quantity, and of good quality.

  Never use expired condoms. You should always check the expiration date printed on the package.

- Store the condoms in a cool, dry place—for example in a drawer by your bed.

- Take the condom out of its wrapping carefully without scratching it with your nails or with your rings and without stretching it.

- A condom should be worn before any intimate relations to avoid catching sexually transmitted diseases.

- Wait until the penis is fully erect. Hold the tip of the condom with your index finger and thumb to prevent air entering, causing it to burst. Leave some space free between the tip of the penis and the condom so that, on ejaculation, the semen is deposited in the receptacle formed by the free space available.

- Place the condom over the tip of the penis without letting go of the end. Peel back the foreskin and roll the condom over the rest of the penis until you reach its base. Use the condom throughout intercourse.

- As soon as ejaculation has occurred, the condom should be removed very slowly. Do not wait to take off the condom until the erection has subsided. When removing it, hold it at the bottom to avoid the semen spilling out.

- After removing it, make a knot in it and throw it into the trash can, never in the toilet.

- Condoms are to be used once only and should therefore never be reused.

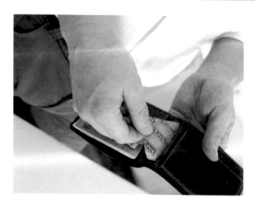

It is not advisable to keep condoms in your billfold or in places that are warm, since heat damages the latex from which the condom is made.

so-called "morning-after pill," as an emergency measure.

- This pill consists of a combination of hormones which alter the menstual cycle. This prevents pregnancy by inhibiting or delaying ovulation and stopping the fertile egg implanting in the lining of the uterus.

- This pill is nearly 100 percent effective, if taken within 24 hours of the condom bursting or other risky situations occurring during sex.

- It should always be taken within 72 hours of having sex and requires a medical prescription.

- The treatment is divided into two doses, the first to be taken within 72 hours of coitus and the second 12 hours after the first dose.

- This method should only be used in case of emergency, not as an alternative form of contraception. For this, there are more effective methods that you can find out about at any family planning center.

- Approximately half of the women who take the morning-after pill experience nausea and, one in five, vomiting. If the vomiting occurs during the two-hour period after taking the pill, the dose should be repeated, since it has still not been absorbed into the bloodstream.

- It must be remembered that the post-coital pill prevents unwanted pregnancy, but it does not protect against sexually transmitted diseases, or against AIDS.

Latex is a milky looking liquid, obtained from the trunk of a tropical tree, the Hevea brasiliensis. After long and complex industrial processing, it is used in the fabrication of rubber and elastics. It is employed in the manufacture of condoms and surgical gloves.

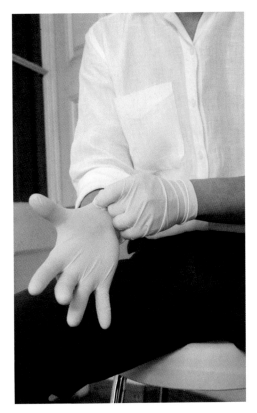

Cases in which the morning-after pill is prescribed

• When the condom bursts or slips off inside the vagina.
• If the couple use natural methods of family planning and have sex during the time of the month when there is a greater risk of pregnancy.
• Because of problems with an IUD (Intrauterine Device).
• Unprotected ejaculation on the external genitals or in the vagina.
• When the daily oral contraceptive has not been taken for more than three consecutive days.
• Rape.

Cases in which the morning-after pill should not be prescribed

• If pregnancy is suspected.
• If unprotected sexual relations have taken place before the risky sexual act in question.

Cases to be assessed by a specialist

• Women who suffer frequent migraines.
• Women who have blood circulation illnesses and alterations in their blood coagulation.
• Women who are breastfeeding their children.
• Women suffering from any illness relating to their reproductive system.

Latex allergy

• Some people, men as well as women, can have allergic reactions when they have sexual relations. This can be caused either by the spermicides used with the condom, or by the latex from which the condom is made.
• To exclude the possibility that the spermicide is causing the allergies, it is advisable to use different brands of spermicide during sexual relations. If the allergic reactions disappear when you change brands, it is quite probable that the allergic reaction is caused by that particular spermicide.
• If the allergic reaction continues or gets worse, consult the doctor who will provide alternative methods of protection.
• There are polyurethane condoms on the market, which reduce the risk of allergic reaction.

How should you react to a sexual assault?

Sexual assaults are acts in which one person, using their physical strength or by means of threats, compels another to have sexual relations against their will. Sexual assaults have physical and mental consequences and they can be committed by strangers, or by people known to the victim. It is necessary to act quickly so that the health services and police may assist the victim and collect the relevant incriminating evidence.

How should you react to a sexual assault?

• Sexual assaults are serious crimes in all developed countries. The first step is to go to the police immediately so that the person who committed the offense can be arrested. This is very important because rapists often re-offend. If you do not

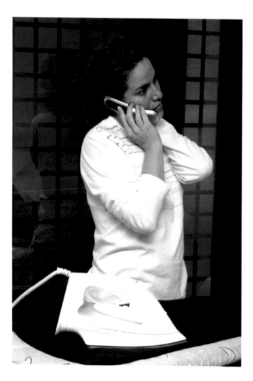

report them to the authorities, it increases the chances of the attacker assaulting another victim.

What to do in the case of a sexual assault

• Try to overcome your torment, anxiety, mistrust, and fear. Try to be calm and remember that you should not remain silent about a sexual assault, whoever the perpetrator may be.

• Call or go to the police. They generally have personnel trained to deal with cases of sexual abuse. During the interview, you will be asked about all the circumstances surrounding the assault (when it happened, how it occurred, in what situation and where). (Under-age victims will be looked after by officers specially trained to deal with minors.) If during the rape, objects were used that were left behind, such as a knife or firearm, etc., these should be handed over to the police.

• Try to remember as much as you can about the attacker and note it down on a piece of paper; describing the clothes and jewelry he was wearing and any other details might help to identify him.

It is very useful to go to the police station accompanied by a person you trust when making your accusations, since it can help you calm down and remember the details and questions you want to ask the authorities.

• When the police have drawn up your statement, read it carefully and sign it. Do not sign it unless you agree completely with what is written down.

• The police authorities will inform you about victims' rights and about support for rape victims.

• You will need a medical examination. Do not change your clothes or shower until the doctor or nurse has finished examining you. Clues may remain on clothing that are indispensable for the investigation. An examination will be conducted: blood samples will be taken and tests performed for evidence of sexually transmitted diseases, unwanted pregnancy, etc., and semen samples will be collected.

• You will also be assessed psychologically to determine what mental trauma has occurred.

• It is advisable for photos to be taken that show all the injuries caused by the attacker; these can be very useful in the event of going to court. Note down with the photos the time and place where each injury was incurred. This is useful for the medical examination by the forensic specialist, since there may have been injuries at the time that have since disappeared.

• Once the forensic specialist has finished the examination, ask for a copy of it. The courts will rely mainly on this report to decide on the appropriate penalty.

**What should you
do if the sexual assault
has taken place within marriage?**

• If you have been sexually assaulted within a stable relationship or within marriage, you should do the following:

• Go to the police so that a statement may be drawn up, and ask for help from the social servic-

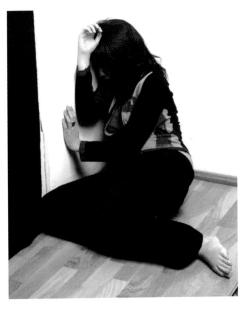

Avoid the enclosed areas of the house, such as the bathroom and corners of rooms where an aggressor can trap his victim.

How to recognize when a child has been sexually assaulted

• The child becomes abnormally afraid of strangers and even his parents, or fears going out into the street.

• Schoolwork goes downhill: lack of concentration.

• Changes in eating habits.

• Changes in sleeping patterns.

• Inappropriate behavior for his age: he may act like an older child or a younger one.

• Self-harming.

• Sexual and aggressive behavior unusual for his age, which comes out in his language, games, and drawings.

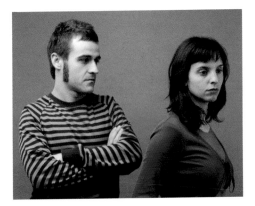

es, who will place you in the hands of a lawyer to assist you and inform you of your rights.

• If the situation has brought a mother and children into danger, they can move out of their home without the wife being accused of wrongfully abandoning the home, or non-fulfillment of her conjugal duties, as long as she has given the police a statement of her accusations against her spouse or partner.

• When abandoning the home, you should collect all documents that could be used as evidence of the conjugal relationship.

• If the lives of the wife and children are at risk, she can ask to be admitted to a refuge.

• If, despite the attacks, the couple continue sharing the home, the following steps should be taken:

• Try to spend most of the time in rooms whose windows and doors are open, or with a telephone, so as to be able to escape, or call for help.

• Keep your cell phone with you at all times.

• Also spend as little time as possible in the kitchen, because knives and other utensils may be used as weapons.

Pedophiles tend to shower their victims with presents so that they feel indebted to the person, and the abuser can thus take advantage of the situation. Children should be taught not to speak to strangers.

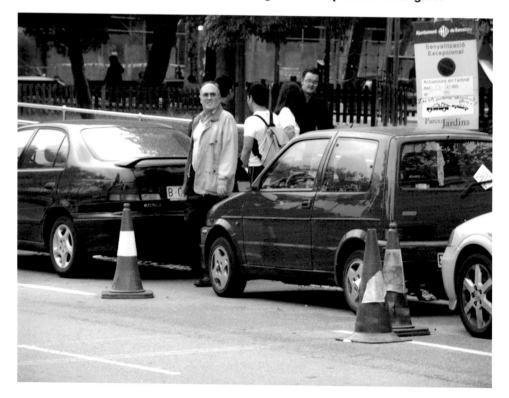

Alcohol poisoning

Alcohol poisoning is the most common type of intoxication in many countries of the world. It can affect people of any sex, age, and social level. Alcohol consumption is responsible for more than half of all road accidents. Furthermore, many people with alcohol problems do not recognize them. It is essential to accept that alcohol is a dangerous drug and, as such, should be consumed responsibly.

Alcohol poisoning

• Alcohol poisoning is caused by the consumption of alcoholic drinks.

• This type of poisoning becomes aggravated when mixed with medications, since it can increase the depressive effect upon the central nervous system and cause death.

• The degree of intoxication depends on the volume consumed, on whether food has been eaten previously, and on the person's tolerance of alcohol.

• The effect produced by drinking two beers is not the same in a person of 200 lb (90kg) who drinks alcohol all the time, as in one of 130 lb (58kg) who almost never drinks.

• Another aspect of alcohol abuse is that it is one of the most common problems among young people and adolescents; it leads them into situations where they have accidents, fights, or unwanted pregnancies. It is therefore important to educate the young about responsible alcohol consumption.

• The main types of alcoholic drinks are the following:

– Fermented drinks. These are based on a grain or fruit and undergo a process of alcoholic fermentation: wine, beer, and cider, etc.

– Distilled drinks. These are produced by distillation of a fermented drink. During the process of

What to do in the case of alcohol poisoning

The following symptoms are signs of severe alcohol poisoning:

• Vomiting.

• Loss of consciousness.

• Shaking.

• If you encounter someone who you know has been drinking alcohol and has these symptoms, you should:

• Take the person to the emergency room, where he will be re-hydrated and given vitamin B6.

• Try to wrap up the victim, as he must not get cold.

• This is important, since people with alcohol poisoning have problems regulating their body temperature.

• If on the way, the poison victim vomits, keep him on his side to prevent him choking on his own vomit.

• Try to keep him awake.

• If the poisoning is not serious, the person will feel extremely unwell and sick. They should be kept hydrated and allowed to rest in a cool, quiet place until the effects of the alcohol have worn off, usually between 12 and 24 hours after the drinking session.

DEGREES OF ALCOHOL POISONING

Degree of poisoning	Alcohol level in the blood	Symptoms
First degree	50–80 mg/100 mL (about three shots of whiskey or 4 beers)	• Lack of coordination • Incessant talking • Euphoria • No sensation of fatigue • Sensation of heightened reflexes
Second degree	80–150 mg/100 mL	• Incessant talking • Impulsiveness • Lack of inhibition • Irritability • Clumsy movement
Third degree	150–400 mg/100 mL	• Aggressive attitude • Confused language • Difficulty in maintaining balance • Possibility of loss of consciousness
Fourth degree	400 mg/100 mL	• Depression of the nervous system • Death

distillation, part of the water content is eliminated, thus increasing the degree of alcohol: whiskey, rum, gin, and tequila, etc.

How alcohol should be enjoyed

- Always drink on a full stomach.
- Drink with the intention of tasting the drink and savoring it, not for the effects of intoxication. This is very important for young people, whose main reason for drinking is to get drunk.
- Mix non-alcoholic drinks with alcoholic ones.
- Do not use drinking as an excuse to forget stressful situations in daily life, as a means of relaxation, or as a tranquilizer. This puts you at risk of

Alcoholism increases the risk of developing cancer of the esophagus, throat, larynx, mouth, and breasts.

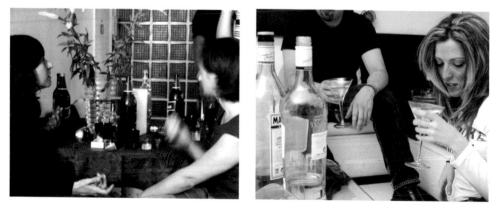

becoming an alcoholic. To get rid of anxiety and stress, it is best to take exercise, to try to rest, or do things together with your loved ones.

• Do not drink and drive.

• Avoid drinking adulterated alcohol.

• Everyone should know their own limits. Controlling the symptoms that alcohol produces in the body and knowing when to stop drinking can prevent many cases of intoxication.

What is drinking in moderation?

• A few years ago, it was demonstrated that moderate alcoholic consumption has a protective effect on the circulatory system. In men, to drink in moderation is to have one or two glasses of wine or beer a day, always at meal times.

• In women, moderate drinking is having one glass of wine or beer a day, always with food. It is best to go without alcohol one day a week.

Alcoholism in women

• Women are more sensitive to alcohol than men, since they have a larger quantity of fatty tissue, a smaller proportion of water and blood in their bodies, and fewer liver enzymes for metabolizing alcohol.

• If a woman and a man consume the same amount of alcohol, the intoxication will be more pronounced in the woman.

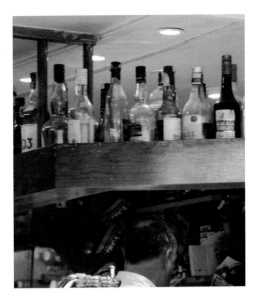

• If consumption takes place over a long period, it has been demonstrated that liver damage is much more serious in women than in men. Alcohol can also cause menstruation problems.

• The social tolerance of excessive drinking by men does not extend to women, causing their alcoholism to develop in a more silent and furtive manner and leading to more cases of alcoholic depression.

Hangover remedies

Hangover symptoms, such as nausea, headaches, acidity in the stomach, and general exhaustion, tend to settle down in approximately 24 hours. The following advice is to enable you to help your body recover after excessive drinking:

• It has been shown that fructose, a sugar found in fruit, helps to eliminate alcohol from the body more quickly. In cases of alcohol intoxication, it is therefore recommended to drink juices made from fruit and honey.

• Drink a lot of water to compensate for the dehydration caused by alcohol.

• Soups and consommés have calming effects on the digestive system and replace lost mineral salts.

• For headaches, it is best to take analgesics orally, such as acetaminophen (Tylenol) or aspirin.

• Rest and sleep for as long as necessary.

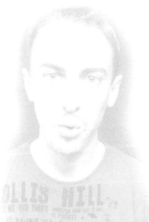

Drug poisoning

The excessive consumption of certain drugs can have effects that may endanger the life of the drug taker. On the other hand, abstaining from drugs suddenly can lead to withdrawal symptoms that seriously affect your health. To combat drugs, you need to know a lot about them and to teach your children how to avoid their use.

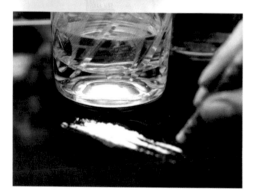

When cocaine is mixed with alcohol, the action of the liver creates a combined substance, called cocaethylene, which intensifies the effects of the cocaine and increases the risk of heart failure.

How to deal with cocaine poisoning

• The signs of cocaine poisoning in a person are the following, depending on the dose taken:
  – Anxiety and worry.
  – Loss of appetite and insomnia.
  – Dilated pupils.
  – Increased heart rate.

Severe cocaine poisoning

• Cocaine is one of the most addictive drugs, especially at a psychological level. Its effects stimulate the central nervous system, causing constriction of the blood vessels, dilation of the pupils, increased heart rate and blood pressure.

• A person who has taken cocaine, especially cocaine hydrochloride via the nasal passage, has symptoms of sleeplessness, no feeling of tiredness, loss of appetite, and an increasing sense of insecurity. It is possible to develop a high tolerance to cocaine, which is why users need increasingly large doses to obtain the desired effects.

Overcoming the heroin withdrawal syndrome lasts about three weeks and breaking the habit completely takes a few months. In the majority of cases, rehabilitation is accompanied by behavioral therapy and psychological support.

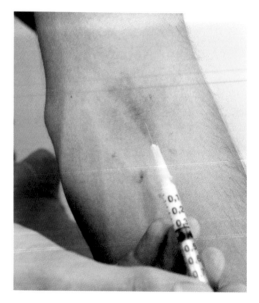

Severe poisoning from LSD and hallucinogens

- Hallucinogenic substances are capable of provoking distortions in perception and the senses, causing hallucinations. The user thinks that these hallucinations are real and in some cases, this can engender panic and real terror.
- Hallucinogenic substances can be found in nature, for example psilocybin, contained in some fungi and mushrooms, and mescaline in the peyote mushroom. Alternatively, they can be synthesized in laboratories in the form of LSD (lysergic acid diethylamide) or PCP (phencyclidine), called "angel dust."

- Users of hallucinogens experience alterations in perception, in the form of visual and auditory hallucinations.
- Poisoning and overdoses are not usually associated with hallucinogenic substances. However, given that hallucinations can cause terror and panic in the user, commonly known as "a bad trip," accidents can occur as a result of such hallucinations.
- The user should therefore be treated calmly, prevented from injuring himself, and kept in a bright place, which inhibits further hallucinations.
- Later, the victim should be taken to the emergency room to receive suitable medication and to prevent complications.

During the hippie movement of the 1960s, it was common for LSD to be synthesized in clandestine laboratories; however, in recent years, its use has diminished.

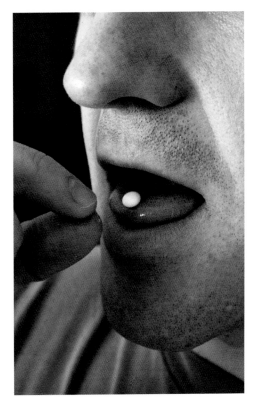

– Raised blood pressure.
– Paleness and nausea.
– Altered consciousness and hallucinations.
– Convulsions and, finally, heart attack.
- Speak to the person calmly, in a low voice, and do not hurry.
- Touch the person gently and explain that their anxiety and nervousness can be treated.
- Take the poison victim to the emergency room so that they can be stomach-pumped and given intravenous medications that reduce the over-stimulation of their central nervous system.

Severe heroin poisoning

- Heroin is a derivative of opium, whose effects are similar to those of morphine, but more intense—that is to say, it is a painkiller that acts as a depressant on the central nervous system.
- Heroin users describe its effects as an absolute sense of well-being, pleasure, heightened powers of imagination, and other sensations that are extremely pleasant.

In the long term, ecstasy causes the same changes to the neurons as Parkinson's disease, inducing shaking and lack of coordination.

• It is a highly addictive drug, which has very severe withdrawal symptoms, consisting of muscle pains, diarrhea, dehydration, alterations in blood composition, and loss of appetite.

How to deal with heroin poisoning

• Patients who have taken an overdose of heroin usually sleep or go into a stupor. They may also fall into a coma. Their breathing rate becomes greatly reduced, and may fall as low as two to four breaths per minute, with their flesh turning a bluish color.

• Body temperature falls and the skin becomes cold and damp.

• If not treated in time, it can lead to death through lung failure.

• Take the poison victim to the emergency room, where he can receive suitable medication and be prevented from going into coma.

• While waiting for medical assistance, you should give pain stimulus to the person, for example by pinching them strongly, since the pain increases the breathing rate and may prevent heart and lung failure.

Severe poisoning from "designer drugs" like ecstasy

• Ecstasy, whose chemical name is methylenedioxymethamphetamine (MDMA), is a drug with properties similar to amphetamines; that is to say, it is hallucinogenic and conducive to intensified social interaction. It also causes increased heart rate and blood pressure, dehydration, and a rise in body temperature.

• Even several weeks after taking it, it can still cause psychological changes, like depression, anxiety, paranoia, and an increase in the desire to take drugs.

What to do if someone is suffering from ecstasy poisoning

• Treat the poison victim calmly and speak to him in a soft, quiet voice.

• If he is suffering from heatstroke, do the following:

— Take him to a cool and gently lit place.

— Cool his body down with wet towels, compresses, or linen, especially on the neck, chest, armpits, and groin.

— Give him cool water, which should be drunk in small sips.

— Take the victim to emergency room to receive suitable medication and to prevent complications.

Cannabis poisoning

• Marijuana is a widely consumed drug, which is obtained from the hemp plant Cannabis sativa and whose main active ingredient is THC (tetrahydrocannabinol).

• The effects of marijuana on the user are usually changes in physical coordination, eye irritation, an increased sense of well-being, and greater appetite. In some cases, it causes fainting.

• If taken regularly, physical tolerance to drugs like cannabis develops and they require an increasing dose to produce the desired effect. They can also lead to psychological dependency that is moderate to severe.

What to do in the case of cannabis poisoning

• The effects of this drug are not considered very dangerous, since physical dependency is slight. However, depending on the amount taken and the health of the user, they can have some harmful effects.

• If you feel slight nausea , become too hot, or faint, it is better to rest. Drink a lot of water; do not become alarmed, keep calm and wait for the bad trip to pass.

• If somebody has symptoms of vomiting, cold sweats, lack of coordination, or loss of consciousness, take him to the nearest hospital.

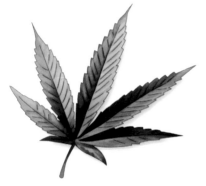

Long-term use of cannabis causes lack of motivation, reduced ability to concentrate, and impaired short-term memory.

Prevention of accidents involving children

When there are children in the home, it is important to change your attitude to the objects in your surroundings. Children's curiosity is unlimited and just as almost any object can be transformed into a toy, it can also become a risk.

Children in the street

• Children must never be left alone or unsupervised in the street. If they have to be left some-

where, this must always be in the care of someone trustworthy.

• From a very early age, they must be taught their full name, the places where their parents

When walking with your baby in a stroller and crossing the street, do not cross with the child in front of you. Always make sure that he is strapped in safely.

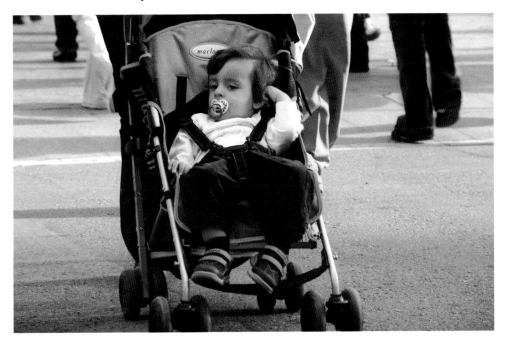

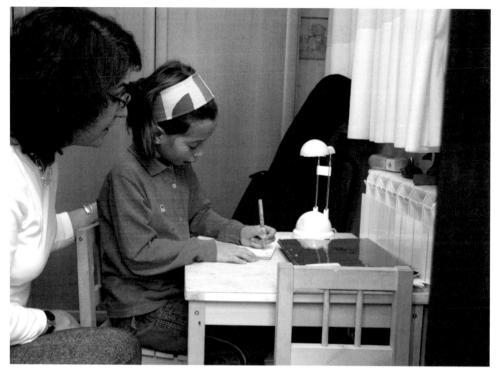

When children are going to spend time alone at home, make sure that they have tasks to carry out—such as school homework or some handwork that they must show the adults when they get home.

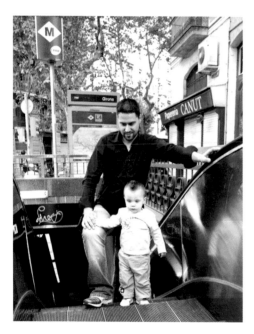

work, and the phone numbers of their home, close family members, and trusted neighbors.

• You must know where your children are at all times. Advise them that when they go out, this should be in a group and in streets frequented by people, avoiding deserted streets.

• When employing someone to look after the children, you should carefully check out all the references they provide.

• It is important to make a list of all the names, surnames, and telephone numbers of the children's friends and keep this somewhere safe.

• Do not allow children to play in abandoned sites or buildings.

• Children should be taught not to talk to strangers and if they come across someone they

Because children do not have a well-developed sense of balance until a certain age, it is best to hold them when going up or down an escalator.

If children stay at home alone

- If for unavoidable reasons, you are forced to leave a child alone at home, the neighbors should be told about it.

- The children should be taught to keep the doors and windows closed, and not to open the door to strangers under any circumstances.

- Children should have a key for getting out of the house that is easy to use.

- Children should be taught never to tell strangers that they are alone in the house.

- It is important to write down a set of instructions for the child on a piece of paper.

- Make sure that they can easily reach the home telephone and that they keep the line free, to allow for incoming calls. A list of emergency telephone numbers should be left next to the phone.

- A child should be taught simple first aid techniques, such as washing cuts and scratches, as well as putting on bandages.

- Before leaving home, verbally go over with the child all the instructions written down on paper, such as not opening the door to strangers, etc.

do not know and who tries to speak to them, they should tell their parents about this.

- Children should be taught not to give their name or address to strangers, not to accept presents, candies, or anything else at all.

- If a child comes home with money or unfamiliar objects, ask how he got them.

- Children should be taught not to keep anything secret from adults.

- From an early age, you should have a good level of communication with children so as to avoid any taboo subjects with them.

- Children should know that when they notice somebody is following them in the street, they

According to statistics, the use of helmets for children has reduced the number of serious head injuries considerably.

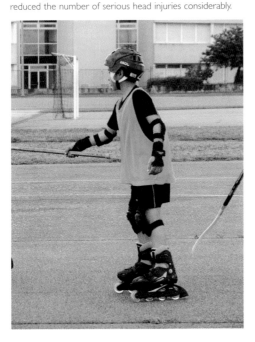

Get a child seat that fulfills all the safety standards and that is officially approved.

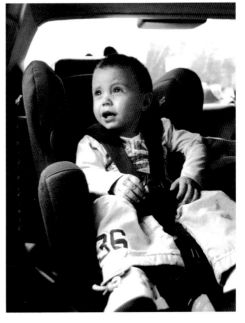

CHILD SAFETY SEATS IN CARS

Weight	Age	How to seat the child
Up to 22 lb (10kg)	Up to 1 year approximately	Opposite to the direction of the car Preferably on a back seat, if possible in the center
From 20 to 40 lb (99 to 18 kg)	From 1 to 3 years old	Forward facing On a back seat, if possible in the center
From 35 to 55 lb (16 to 25 kg)	From 3 to 8 years old	Booster seats on back seats compatible with the seatbelt
From 50 to 80 lb (23 to 36 kg)	From 8 to 12 years old	Booster seat or specially designed cushions until large enough for adult seatbelt to fit correctly

should go into a public place, such as a shop, or into a police station, if there is one nearby.

• A child must get used to obeying all the traffic regulations; for example, only to cross a street when the sign says "Walk."

• Small children tend to run about quickly, so it is advisable to always hold their hands when walking in the street.

• Never allow your child to swim alone in ponds, swimming pools, or other places filled with water, not even when the child knows how to swim and the water is shallow.

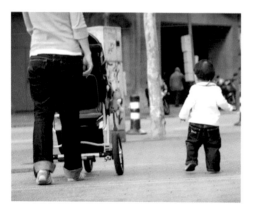

Children in the supermarket or large stores

• Supermarkets are not suitable places for children, but often they have to accompany adults there, on a shopping trip, when no responsible person is available to look after them.

• The child should be taught that supermarkets are not play areas and they shouldn't touch the goods on display.

• If the supermarket or store has an escalator, do not let them play on it and certainly do not allow them to use it unaccompanied by an adult. Escalators carry many dangerous risks, such as falling from one level to another or trapping feet or hands on the side walls.

• Supermarket carts do not meet the safety standards necessary for children to ride on them. If you let your child get on the cart, there is a risk that he will try to reach something on the shelves, with the danger that it might fall on him, causing injury. There is a high risk that the object will fall on his head, or that it might be made of glass and cut him.

• Never leave a child alone in a supermarket; children have often been abducted in supermarkets.

• Even if you are with him, do not let your child run down the aisles, because of the risk of him col-

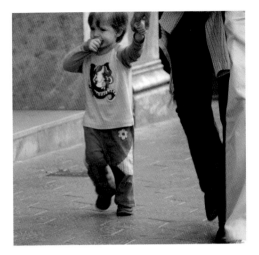

liding with a cart and getting injured. Also, he might get hold of some toxic product, open it, and swallow it.

Children and toys with wheels

• All children should wear safety helmets when riding a bicycle, skateboarding, or roller skating. This is very important, since if they fall over, no matter how serious the fall, the head tends to be the first part of the child to get hit.

• Children under five should not be allowed to ride bicycles alone, especially at dusk or at night, since a quarter of all bicycle accidents happen at this time.

• Get a bicycle that is the right size for the child. He should be able to touch the ground with his feet. To avoid damage and injuries to the genitals, there should be a gap of about an inch (3 cm) between the seat and his groin when he is standing over the stationary bicycle with his feet on the ground.

How to persuade a child to put on his safety helmet

• From the very first moment that a child begins to ride on a bicycle, even if he rides on a little seat behind the adult, he should get accustomed to wearing a helmet. In this way, a habit is built up.

• Adults should set an example by wearing helmets too. Children tend to imitate their parents' behavior.

• The child should be taught that a bicycle is not a toy, but a means of transport and that he should therefore take appropriate safety precautions.

Child walkers can cause accidents by allowing the child to move around faster, which can make a fall down the stairs more probable.

• Explain to the child that falling from a bicycle is dangerous and can be very serious.

• Show him photographs of professional cyclists in helmets.

• Show your appreciation when your child puts on his helmet voluntarily.

• Be firm in your decision about using a helmet and do not allow him to make any journey without it, however short.

• Tell him that if he does not want to use a helmet, he should use another means of transport, rather than a bicycle.

Children in the car: child seats

• The great majority of injuries caused by car accidents can be avoided by using a special seat for children.

• When children travel in a suitable seat for their size, they feel more secure and their behavior is more controllable. The driver, by not having to worry about the child's unpredictable movements, can concentrate more on driving.

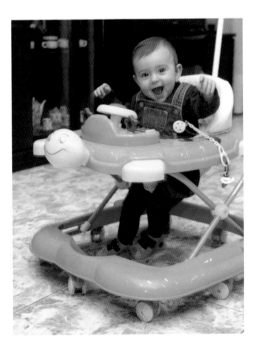

• If you have doubts about how to install the child seat, call the manufacturer for the relevant information.

• The child seat should always be used, even if only driving for a few minutes or a few yards.

When children are under six months old

• Babies tend to be very curious and you should therefore take extra precautions at home, to make sure that everything is adapted for babies.

• At this age, accidents usually occur as a result of parents' carelessness, in not being aware that the child is trying to get out of its cot, or in the kitchen where they have taken the child when they have gone to get a cup of hot coffee.

• To prevent falls when changing diapers, place the baby in a safe place where he cannot fall. This is particularly important when the child reaches the age at which he can turn over by himself.

Adolescents

• Adolescents can have as many or more problems than young children and these problems can be difficult to resolve.

• You should try to keep communicating with the child; then, if problems occur, the adolescent will probably be prepared to talk about them with you. Give time to the child and do some activity with him that he enjoys.

• When a child goes out of the house, you should know who he is going to see and where he is going. It is important to know who his friends are.

• If he rides a moped, make sure he uses a safety helmet.

• Give children clear and full information about all subjects relating to sexuality and contraceptive methods. The more information you give them and the more confidence they gain, the less they will be at risk of unwanted pregnancies and of catching a sexually transmitted disease.

• If the baby is already crawling, the stairway should be protected with a rail and rooms you do not want the baby to go in should have their doors locked.

• Fasten the windows of the house well to avoid the possibility of the child leaning out of them.

• Never eat or drink hot foods in front of the baby, since he might make an effort to reach them and burn himself; this is especially important when holding the baby in your arms.

• Do not leave any objects that he can put in his mouth within reach of the baby.

• Do not give solid foods to the child, which might cause choking.

• Cover the household electric sockets with protectors to avoid electrical accidents.

• If the house has stairs, protective gates should be installed on them.

• Lock up cleaning products and medications. If they are kept in a high place, this can cause the baby to fall when he tries to climb up to reach them. Keep a list by the phone of useful telephone numbers in case of a poisoning emergency.

When school has finished

• When the child gets home after school, he should be carefully supervised, especially in small families when there is only one family member looking after him.

• If it is not possible to manage the household tasks and watch over the child at the same time, you should employ somebody to help you look after your child.

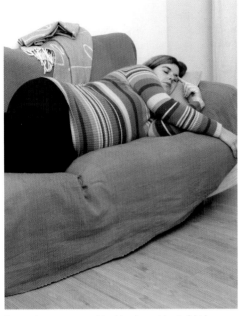

Pregnant women are advised to sleep at least eight hours a day and, if possible, should also have a siesta.

six principal nutritional groups, that is to say: meat, vegetables, fruit, cereals, eggs, and dairy products. Healthy nutrition should be based on these six fundamental elements. Otherwise, there will be a lack of essential nutrients and this could harm the fetus's development. The idea of variety must apply to each group, so, for example, in the case of dairy products, she should consume milk, yogurt, and all types of cheese, etc., to ensure an intake of all the essential nutrients.

The idea of quantity does not mean eating for two, as is generally thought. It is based on eating the necessary quantities of each type of food and not eating too much, or too little.

Pregnant women's sleep problems

• Pregnant women often have problems sleeping while the fetus continues to grow inside them.

• They can also have particular problems in the first three months of pregnancy, due to the unpleasant symptoms in their breasts and the generalized discomfort associated with the first few months.

• The recommended position for sleeping is lying on your left side, since this position is favorable for the blood circulation. In this way, the appearance of hemorrhoids and stomach and digestive complications can be avoided.

• Pregnant women should not take sleeping medications; this type of treatment is completely contraindicated.

• It is advisable to use natural remedies for getting to sleep, such as having a glass of hot milk before sleeping and practicing relaxation techniques.

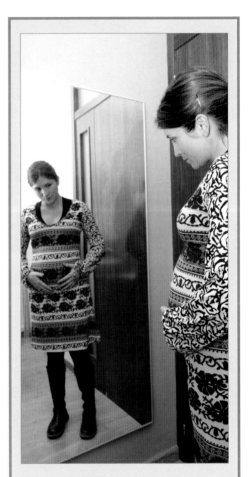

How do you recognize a contraction?

• Touch your abdomen.

• If you can push your finger toward the inside, it means that the uterus is still relaxed.

• If, on the other hand, the surface is hard and firm, you are having a contraction.

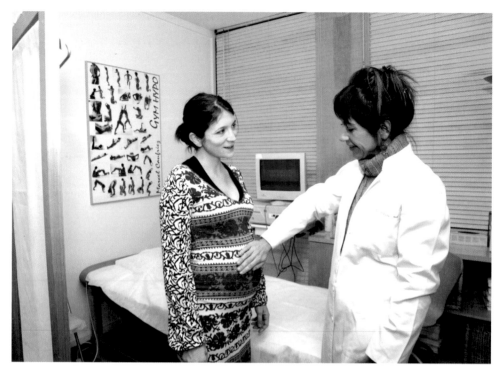

Women who decide to get pregnant after the age of 35 should undergo a full medical examination, to detect and treat possible health problems.

Mothers over 35

• Nowadays, women delay pregnancy because their priorities have changed; for example, they may want to wait until they have achieved their professional goals.

• As a result, the number of women who become pregnant after the age of 35 has increased considerably.

• In general, it is not the age of the pregnant mother that is important, but rather her state of

Suggestions for mothers over the age of 35

• Before getting pregnant, go to the gynecologist and tell him you plan to get pregnant. If you are in one of the risk groups, he will do some analysis and tests to check on your state of health.

• Ask for regular and frequent checkups during pregnancy.

• Ask for prenatal tests to rule out abnormalities in the fetus.

• Follow the other recommendations for younger pregnant women—that is to say, not smoking, not drinking alcohol, not taking drugs and, before taking any medication, consulting the specialist.

• Maintain a diet that is balanced in variety and quantity. Eat foods that are rich in folic acid, such as cereals. It is proven that taking folic acid reduces the risk of fetal malformations in the central nervous system.

Stress has more effect on the ability to get pregnant than on the pregnancy itself. A couple under stress will have less chance of a pregnancy than if they are calm and relaxed.

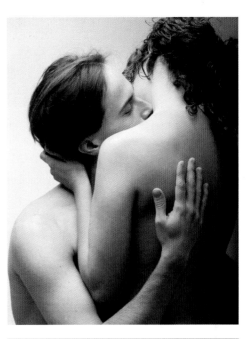

health during the years before she became pregnant.

• After the age of 30, women as well as men are more prone to suffer chronic illnesses, such as diabetes, high blood pressure and heart problems. These illnesses can make pregnancy problematic.

• Thus, women who decide to get pregnant after the age of 35 need to undergo more exhaustive checkups than younger women during pregnancy, to prevent complications for the mother, as well as the fetus.

How does stress affect the mother?

• Women who are stressed during pregnancy suffer the same consequences as the rest of the population.

• Stress produces a discharge of epinephrine (adrenaline), constriction of the blood vessels and even contractions of the uterus, although this does not constitute a risk for the mother or the fetus.

Should pregnant women drive?

• Pregnant women are recommended to drive as little as possible during the last months of pregnancy, although this advice is simply because of the discomfort of sitting inside the vehicle. If she decides to drive till the last day of her pregnancy, there is no risk involved, since she will be quite capable of driving.

• Seatbelts are obligatory for pregnant women just as they are for any other citizen, but have increased importance in that they are there also to protect the unborn child.

Sex and pregnancy

• Many women wonder if they can have sex during pregnancy and if this can affect the fetus in any way. Each trimester of pregnancy brings some new sexual changes that you must be aware of. However, in certain situations, the pregnant mother should consult the doctor before having sex:

– If she bleeds after sexual relations.

– If she has uterine contractions after sex.

Can pregnant women be vaccinated?

• Currently, there is no conclusive evidence regarding risk to the fetus when the mother is vaccinated.

• When a woman is pregnant and exposed to risks of infection, in getting vaccinated, she runs a much smaller risk of harming the fetus than she would if she contracted an infectious illness that spread to the fetus.

• However, when the vaccination is composed of living viruses, its administration to pregnant women is contraindicated, since the living virus can transfer to the placenta and infect the fetus. This situation may occur if the mother is vaccinated in error, or if she is vaccinated without knowing she is pregnant. In this event, she should go immediately to the gynecologist for information regarding possible risks to the fetus and the appropriate measures to take. In the great majority of the cases, it is not necessary to interrupt the pregnancy.

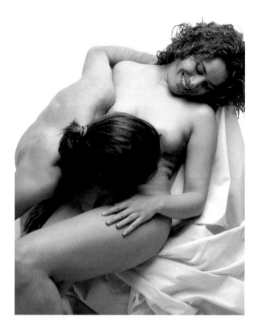

The upper belt should be placed between the breasts of the woman and the lower belt over the thighs, leaving it loose below the abdomen to avoid discomfort and, if there is a sharp pull, when braking suddenly, the force is not concentrated on the abdomen.

The most likely scenario is that at night, the woman will want to rest in bed and sleep peacefully.

• Furthermore, the increase in the size of her breasts make them more sensitive during these first three months, so that she will not be very receptive to the caresses of her partner, since the slightest touch is likely to cause her pain. However, in women with small breasts, it has an opposite effect, since the increase in their breast's size make them more attractive to their partner and their libido increases. Whatever the case, any stimulation of the breasts should be extremely gentle.

• In some women, especially if they have had miscarriages, sexual contact can produce anxiety, since they see it as a threat to the fetus.

– If she has a history of premature birth.

– After she has undergone a prenatal test, such as amniocentesis or chorionic villus sampling.

– If the woman has repeated contractions throughout the day.

Can sexual relations induce birth?

• It is usual to recommend sexual abstinence during the last six weeks of gestation. However, this recommendation has no scientific basis, so that if a couple so desire, they can continue sexual relations as long as they want to, but only if the mother and her partner are comfortable and feel like it.

• The female orgasm, despite causing uterine contractions, does not induce birth, nor does it represent any danger to the fetus.

• It is also often pointed out that semen contains a substance called "prostaglandin," which is used to induce births. Semen in contact with the uterus could thus in theory induce a premature birth. But this notion is questionable, since the quantity of prostaglandin is so small that it could not possibly induce birth.

Sex during the first trimester

• A woman who has just got pregnant and who has symptoms of nausea and vomiting, does not feel particularly receptive to sexual relations, especially if the nausea continues throughout the day.

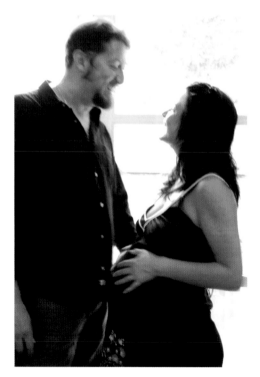

Can a woman do some physical activity during pregnancy?

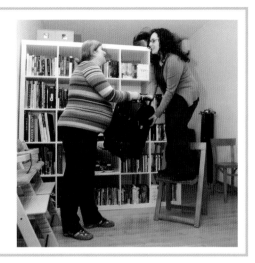

- In general, no particular physical activity is contraindicated, as long as it is done in a moderate way and the woman's body is accustomed to doing it.

- It is not recommended for the pregnant woman to spend a long time standing, or that she should try to take up new sports.

Pregnant women are not advised to lift heavy objects.

Sex during the second trimester

- In this phase of pregnancy, the woman is usually more receptive to sex than in the earlier months, since her nausea and vomiting will probably have disappeared. It is the time to try out comfortable positions for the mother and father.

Sex during the third trimester

- During this period of pregnancy, the mother can start to feel unpleasant symptoms again in her stomach area as well as acidity, due to the pressure of the fetus on the stomach.

- Other complaints may be of a psychological nature, since pregnant women tend to see themselves as larger than they really are and to think that these drastic changes cannot be exciting for their partner. In fact, the reality is sometimes very different, since many fathers find these changes to their wife's body attractive.

▟ Advice for overcoming nausea

- It is better to have little snacks during the day rather than a few heavy meals, since the nausea can get worse if the stomach is empty.

- If you take vitamin tablets during pregnancy, consult a specialist, since some preparations can cause nausea.

- Avoid eating food that is very hot or spicy, fried or very fatty, since this can produce acidity and stomach discomfort.

- Some pregnant women experience less nausea when they eat yogurt or have tea with lemon.

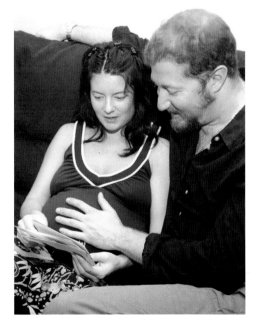

Accident prevention at home

Accidents in the home are usually minor, but if you total them all up, including burns, electric shocks, and small house fires, the level of risk in the home is clearly significant. As in every case, the best way to deal with these types of accidents is by means of prevention.

In the kitchen

The kitchen is one of the most dangerous places in the house: there is a very high risk of serious burns from hot liquids and food.

Whenever you are going to handle containers that are very hot, always use oven mitts, especially when taking food out of the oven when it is still on.

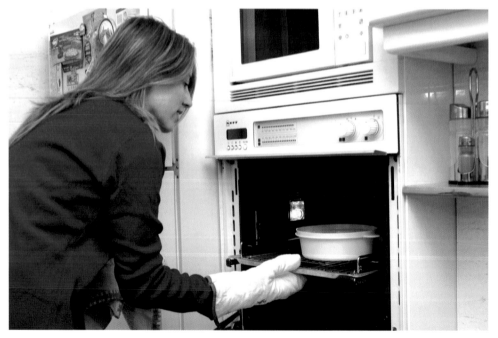

Avoiding burns in the kitchen

• If you are cooking in the presence of small children, keep them away from areas close to the stove and oven and make them sit in a special place.

• If a child can already walk, he will tend to open all the doors within reach, which is why there is a danger of him opening the door of the hot oven; for this reason, you should keep a child away from these areas while you are cooking.

• It is also important not to leave containers that have hot liquids or food in them, for example, hot cups of coffee and pans, within the reach of children.

• Saucepan handles should be directed inward, toward the wall, to prevent hot pans falling. The handles of pots and pans should be made from insulating materials. Whenever you are going to use oil in saucepans, put on a lid that fits the pan, not too large or too small.

• Electrical appliances that produce heat, like toasters, should be kept high up, out of the reach of children. Remember also to keep the cables of appliances out of reach.

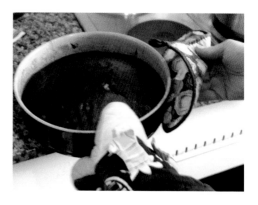

• Remove all lighters from the house to avoid children playing with them.

• Never cook with a child in your arms, since in giving your attention to the child and the food at the same time, there is a greater risk of careless lapses, which could cause accidents, like burns.

• In the case of a burn, the affected area should be placed immediately under water for at least

Check that the smoke detectors are free of dust and other particles that might impair their functioning.

Regarding smoke detectors

• There are some very reasonable smoke detectors on the market. If you place them in appropriate places, you will give yourself some peace of mind.

• These smoke detectors work on batteries that should be replaced once a year at least. Do not forget to do this, since if not, the detector will be completely useless.

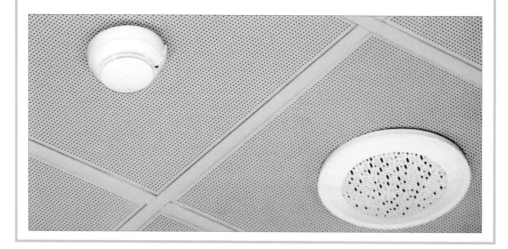

10 minutes and then covered with a sterile dressing.

Make an emergency plan for the home

• It is very useful to make an escape plan for fires in the home, since this is a situation in which it is very easy to allow yourself to be overcome by panic.

• Talk to the children and ask them questions like: how would you escape from a fire? It is advisable to speak to the family about how they would escape from their rooms in case of fire. If you can plan two different ways of getting out of the rooms, the plan will be much more effective.

• Show the family members what they should do during a fire and explain to them that they must keep low and stay as near the ground as possible, because smoke tends to rise toward the roof, leaving oxygen you can breathe near the ground.

Preventing people falling

• At home, falls are often caused by the floor not being clean, with oily patches on them or remains of water used for cleaning. Another cause is when the floor is slippery, due to over-waxing.

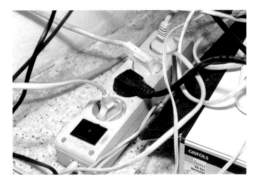

Decide on the safest place in the house and make sure the rest of the family remember it; in the event of fire, all family members should meet there to escape.

• Falls also often occur from windows or balconies with low rails.

• Situations like changing a bulb, standing on a chair, instead of using a suitable step-ladder, also cause injuries.

• To avoid unnecessary falls, follow the steps below:

– Do not use carpets and if you do, try to fix them down well to the floor, especially at the edges.

– Avoid placing obstacles on the floor, especially in the corridors and other places you usually pass through. Pick up the children's toys and those of the pets, too.

– Illuminate the household areas people pass through well, like the corridors and stairs.

– Avoid waxed floors; the floor should be clean, but not slippery.

– At home, wear comfortable and adjustable rubber-soled slippers.

– If you live with elderly people, install handgrips near the toilet, the bathtub, and other necessary places. You should also install a light switch by the bedside to prevent the elderly person wandering about in the dark.

– The stairs should always have a handrail, whose minimum height should be 3 feet (90 cm).

– Check the height of the upstairs windows. If they are less than 3 feet (1 meter) from the floor, install protective measures, such as grilles or rails, to prevent people falling.

– The windows should have safety devices that prevent them being opened by children.

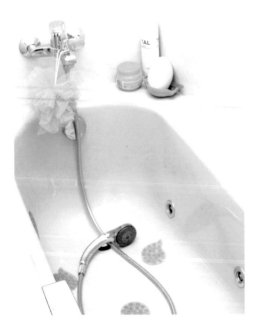

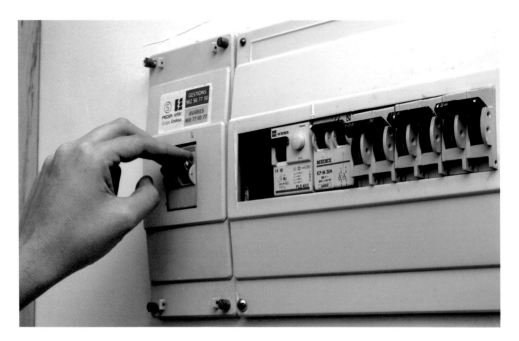

Whenever you are going on vacation, check all the electric and gas appliances, and shut off the supply.

— Shelves should be well fixed to the wall to prevent them collapsing.

— Prevent children from getting up onto the tables, sofas, and other furniture.

— Do not suspend flowerpots on balconies or other objects from the railings.

Safety regarding chemical products and medications at home

• Accidents at home involving the ingestion of chemical products can be very serious. You should therefore follow certain safety rules to avoid accidents with medications, insecticides, cleaning products and solvents, etc.

• Cleaning products should be kept locked up. If this is not possible, they should be kept out of sight and out of reach of children. If they are left in a place that is difficult to reach, but in sight, children might be attracted by the colors of the containers and try to climb up to them, which might cause them to fall.

• Before using any cleaning product, insecticide, or toxic substance, it is necessary to read the instructions on the container carefully. Do not mix cleaning products. For example, when you mix bleach and hydrochloric acid (found in various cleaning products), it produces highly toxic gases. In the case of insecticides, these should not be used on food or domestic animals. If you are going to use insecticide in an enclosed place, you should spray, then close the room and wait some time before going back in. When you re-enter, air the place by opening the doors and windows.

• Medications should be kept locked up and should not be stored in bedside cupboards.

• When painting the house, this should be done with doors and windows open to assist ventilation, especially if you have to use solvents. When you have finished painting the house, do not stay in it until the smell of paint has disappeared.

Avoiding gas poisoning at home

Carbon monoxide (CO) poisoning is to blame every year for some fatal accidents. It is essential to follow certain guidelines when using gas appliances and dealing with gas leaks, if you want to avoid more harmful consequences.

• Avoid using braziers, due to the fire risk. Gas stoves should never be placed in enclosed places without ventilation. When using them, always have the window half open, which will allow the rooms in the house to be ventilated.

• Never have the car's motor running in the garage. If you are going to start up, open the garage door and windows.

• Do not put gas heaters in the bathroom, but choose instead a well-ventilated area in the house.

• If you smell gas inside the house, do not light any kind of naked flame or turn electric switches on or off.

■ How to avoid domestic injuries

• Little cuts and wounds are very common in all homes and are usually caused by careless lapses, such as leaving knives and scissors in the reach of children, and not disposing of containers with sharp edges correctly, such as opening food cans and leaving them in sight, etc.

• Cutting or puncturing your skin can be avoided by following a series of steps:

• Keep all household knives and sharp objects locked up.

• When using knives, scissors, needles, and other items that can injure you, put them back in a locked place after using them to prevent them being accessible.

• Do not have prickly plants as decorations in the house.

• In the kitchen, check damaged plates and glasses regularly.

Toxic products should be kept in their original containers, and should not be swapped round. If you do decide to change containers, make sure you label them well. Avoid transferring toxic cleaning products to containers of consumable products, such as drinks bottles or food jars.

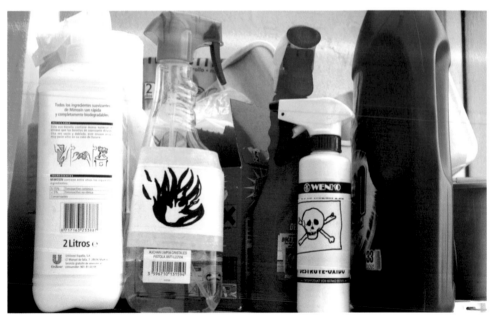

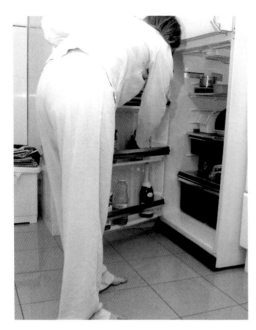

Do not connect or disconnect electrical appliances in your bare feet.

Put bright stickers on large glass windows and doors to avoid people walking into them.

How to avoid accidents with objects at home

Knocks in the home generally occur when you collide accidentally with certain household objects, like furniture, windows, chairs, sofas, and shelving, etc. To avoid these knocks, all these fittings and objects should be kept in perfect order and well secured to avoid them moving accidentally:

- Make an exhaustive check of anything in the house you might hit accidentally, especially those in areas that people pass through frequently, like corridors.

- Open and shut the doors to check their radius of movement and make sure people do not have to pass within these areas.

- Keep all tools and heavy objects in secure places, locked up if possible.

- Check all the household furniture and move those items that stick out or have sharp edges. When furnishing the house, choose items that have rounded edges.

- Do not hang flowerpots on balconies. Always place them at ground level behind the railings.

- Whenever you open a drawer, always close it again. Put stoppers on the drawers, to avoid them falling on people who open them.

- Secure the household shelving well to prevent it falling on the occupants of the house.

How to prevent electrocution

All homes constitute an electrocution risk, simply because they have electrical appliances. The 120 volt domestic supply of any home can cause death. The most common accidents though, are shocks.

- To prevent these dangerous accidents, you should not walk barefoot around the house. This is especially important in rooms that usually contain electrical appliances and have a damp atmosphere, such as the bathroom and kitchen. The risk is compounded if the floor is wet and you go around barefoot.

- The following advice should help to prevent electrocution and electrical accidents at home:

- Electrical appliances in the bathroom should be as far as possible from the bathtub and basin to avoid getting splashed by water. If, despite these precautions, the appliance has come into contact with water, do not connect it until it is completely dry.

- Put child protectors on all the household wall sockets.

Accident prevention on vacation

Admissions to hospital increase during the vacation period due to food poisoning, burns, sunstroke, and injuries caused by road accidents. When on vacation, you should avoid taking risks, so as to be able to return to daily life with renewed vitality.

Avoiding sunburn

Sunburn occurs as a result of overexposure to the damaging ultraviolet rays of the sun. Although the symptoms are normally temporary, skin damage is often permanent and long-term severe effects on your health may occur.

• It is advisable to leave the house with your sunblock already applied and to repeat applications if you swim, even though the sunblock may

Children should use total-protection sunblock, which prevents the sun's harmful rays penetrating to the deepest layers of their skin, which has still not developed all the necessary barriers in the epidermis against sunshine.

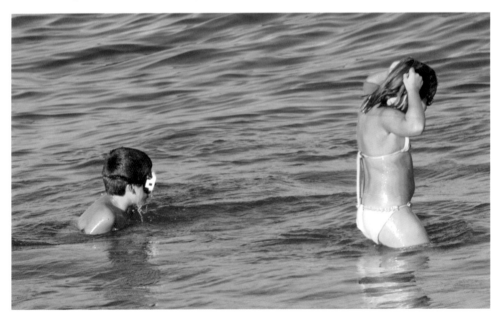

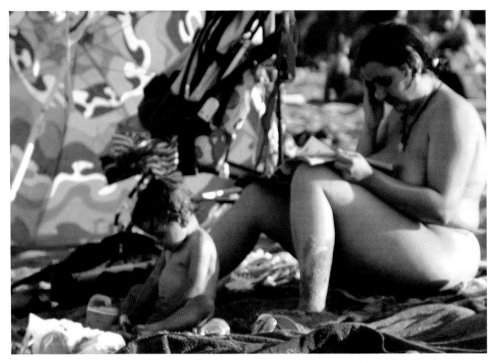

It is recommended to drink a minimum of 2 liters of liquid a day, in the from of water, milk, and juices, etc.

be water-resistant, since drying off and sand make the sunblock less effective.

• Sunbathing should be done progressively. In the early morning, it is not advisable to receive direct sunlight for more than 10 minutes, so you should increase exposure little by little. The recommended procedure is to sunbathe progressively, 5 minutes more each time.

• Children under six months should not be exposed to the sun unless they are covered with some light-colored clothing, even if they are protected under a hat.

How to avoid dehydration

• To avoid dehydration and heatstroke, children taken to the beach should wear light and pale-colored clothing that they can take off easily.

• Avoid exposure to the sun between 11am and 4pm, since the sun's rays are more intense during that time and cause dehydration.

• Eat food containing a lot of water, like salads.

• If you feel nausea, stop what you are doing and rest for a few minutes with a cool drink.

How to avoid sunstroke

• At the beach, in addition to burns, one of the most dangerous effects of the sun is sunstroke.

• Sunstroke is caused by excessive, unprotected exposure to the sun.

• To prevent this, you should take the following advice:

• Do not sunbathe between 11am and 4pm.

• If you must expose yourself to the sun, cover your head with a hat or cap and stay in the sun for as short a time as possible.

• During the period when the sun is strongest, do not play sports and keep unnecessary physical effort to a minimum.

• If you are going to be in the sunshine, use high-factor sunscreen.

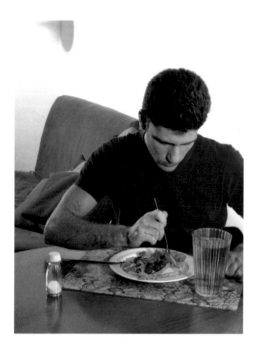

During the journey, the driver should avoid heavy meals and the consumption of alcohol. Fried, spicy, or very salty foods are not recommended either. Large meals tend to cause drowsiness. Go for salads and light meals that are easy to digest. To drink, it is best to have fresh water, juices, and soft drinks that are not carbonated.

Avoiding complications when traveling by car

Before the journey

• Before setting off, get a mechanic to check your car over completely. Get all the maintenance done that has been delayed so far that year—checks such as the brake fluid, oil, water, tires, and make sure you have replacement bulbs, etc.

• When you decide on the itinerary, look for a route that is the most suitable one for the driver. Starting off first thing in the morning helps to avoid those typical vacation traffic jams. Leaving a couple of days before or after the date of the vacation exodus also helps to avoid getting stuck in heavy traffic.

• If you are going to exercise during the hottest period, you will need to hydrate yourself before beginning the activity and continue hydrating during the exercise, drinking something cool roughly every 20 minutes.

• Avoid strenuous exercise altogether during the hottest hours. The best time for exercise is early in the morning or late in the evening.

• If the car does not have air-conditioning, it is best not to travel in the middle of the day, since it may get too hot. Furthermore, excessive heat makes the driver get drowsy and tired.

• If you are driving east, avoid traveling at dawn so that the sun is not in the driver's eyes. If, on the other hand, you are driving west, avoid driving at dusk for the same reason.

• You should only begin the journey when the driver feels rested and in a perfect state of health. Drowsiness is a danger that often causes accidents, because shutting your eyes even for few seconds can lead to a collision.

• Children should sit in the back seat, whatever their age.

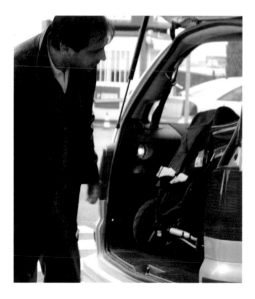

When loading the trunk, this should be done in a sensible orderly way. That is to say, the load should be spread uniformly. Do not put cases or objects in the rear of the car if they are likely to impair the visibility of the driver when looking in the rearview mirror.

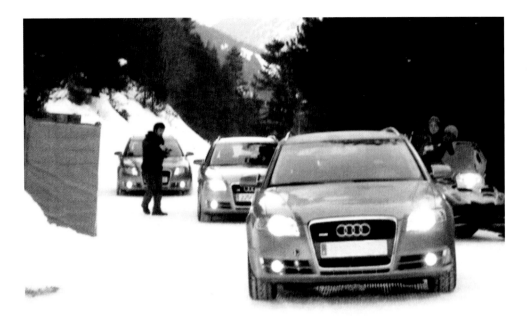

• Before starting the journey, if you do not have specially approved child seats, go to a specialist shop where they will recommend the most suitable type of seat for the child's age.

• Before leaving, if you have children, check how to adjust their special seats. They may have grown since your last trip and you will have to adjust the seats accordingly.

During the journey

• A great many accidents are caused by not respecting the traffic signs. Remember that driving in a law-abiding manner reduces the chances of an accident.

• You should pay special attention to the speed limits for each type of road: These limits can be reduced in the case of construction work and other traffic problems. Always be alert to the speed limits.

• Making regular stops during the journey is recommended, perhaps every 100 to 120 miles (160 to 200 km) or every two hours. Never drive for longer than eight hours each day.

• If you are going to drive on the backroads, adjust your speed accordingly. Many accidents tend to occur on these roads because drivers often drive as though they were on a highway.

• It is a mistake to think that driving carefully can endanger other road users.

On a car journey, it is advisable to give children toys that are officially approved for their age. Avoid toys with sharp edges, which could hurt them if the car brakes suddenly. For example, instead of giving them pencils and ballpoints, wax crayons would be better.

• Stay calm at all times. If the car gets into a jam, take it philosophically and help the rest of the family not to get impatient. Impatience always causes additional problems when driving.

• When you set off, do not calculate what time you are going to pass each point on the journey, or what time you are going to arrive at your destination. Such thoughts always lead to hurrying and anxiousness, which tend to be translated into reckless driving.

• The driver should wear loose comfortable clothing. It is best not to try out new clothing on a long car journey. Your footwear should also be comfortable, with a sole that does not slip when touching the car pedals; thus, for example, driving in beach sandals is not recommended.

• It is not advisable for the driver to smoke during the journey. Tobacco is distracting, when lighting a cigarette, when smoking, and when

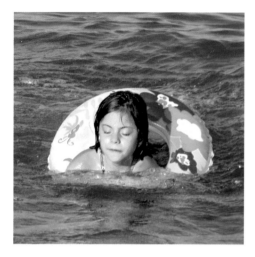

It is not advisable for children to use inflatable rings around their waists to keep afloat, since their effectiveness is not assured in case of drowning. The best solution is the type of floats that are strapped to their bodies, which allow them to move their hands and feet, helping them learn how to swim. Inflatable arm bands are also good for giving a child confidence in the water.

putting it out. Besides, if the windows are kept shut, the smoky atmosphere can make driving difficult.

• If you have children, when you get a car, make sure that the doors have child safety locks to prevent them being opened when the car is in motion.

• It is dangerous for a mother to travel in a car with a child in her arms, both secured by one seatbelt. Avoid this kind of unsafe arrangement.

• When arriving at your destination, do not forget to turn off the motor and the lights, and to put the parking brake on.

How to prevent drowning in pools, beaches, and lakes

• Many schools and nurseries offer the possibility of enrolling young children in swimming courses. They teach infants to float in the water, and later they teach them to swim.

• When they bathe, children should always have an accompanying adult, even in shallow water. Children might begin to swallow water and choke, even if they are touching the bottom of the pool with their feet. Never leave them alone.

• While you are supervising their bathing, prevent them from doing things like fighting or pushing other children underwater.

• If you are taking children out in a boat, they should be equipped with life jackets that they should try out before getting on the boat, to check that they are suitable for their height and weight.

• If your home has a pool and the children still do not know how to swim, it should have a protective railing at least 4 feet high (1.2 meters) to make sure they cannot climb over it. You should not install gates in the fence, in case children are able to open them and fall into the pool.

• Set an example to the children by avoiding bathing in areas with a "bathing not permitted" sign, or where the water has strong currents. If an adult does not respect these instructions, neither will the children.

• Children should be taught the meaning of the beach flags and how they should behave when bathing, according to each flag's color.

• If the children are adolescents and you suspect they have consumed alcohol, under no circumstances allow them to go into the water, not even if it is a pool.

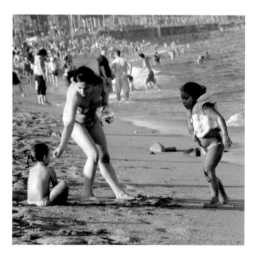

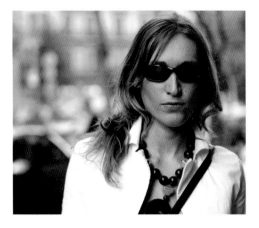

How can you prevent eye injuries in summer?

• During the summer vacations, exposure of the eyes to sunlight increases, as do open-air activities, which can lead to an increased risk of eye injuries.

• Eye injuries in summer are easy to avoid by protecting your eyes and looking after them when engaged in risky activities.

• Use protective glasses whenever you are going to play any open-air sport; there is a very high risk of being hit in the eye by a tennis, squash, or golf ball, which will involve an immediate visit to the emergency room.

• You should also use protective eyeglasses if you are keen on do-it-yourself home improvements or gardening, since, while you are doing these activities, little twigs, splinters and other objects can penetrate the eyeball, causing injuries that may prove very severe.

• When going to the beach, use officially approved sunglasses, bought from the optician, who can give advice on the most suitable type of lenses for the activity you need them for. If you are a sailing enthusiast, it is best to use polarized lenses that help to filter the ultraviolet rays from the sunlight and reflections from the water.

• When swimming in a pool, always wear appropriate swimming goggles that help to reduce the eye irritation caused by contact with the pool water. This usually contains chlorine that often causes stinging in the eyes.

• If you feel you have a foreign body in your eye, do not rub it, because this can make the situation worse, causing very troublesome abrasions to the eyeball. If there is some sand in your eye, put your eye under the water from a faucet until the irritation has disappeared.

• Do not forget your regular visit to the ophthalmologist, so as to rule out any possible eye conditions, problems with vision, and infections that might get worse during the vacation season.

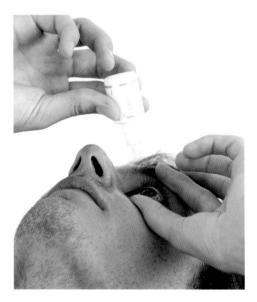

Wearing sunglasses protects you from sand and other particles carried by the wind that might get into your eyes, causing dryness and irritation. If the dryness is very uncomfortable, you can consult the pharmacist to get eye drops and artificial tears that help to keep your eyes in a perfect state of hydration.

Accident prevention at work

In most workplaces, basic accident prevention procedures are carried out in some form or another. There are rules on how materials should be moved, about care in the use of specific work surfaces, order and cleanliness in the workplace, fire prevention, and the use of electricity. However, experience shows that, even though we try to prevent them, accidents do happen at work. Thus, even if you have the best of plans for the prevention or control of operational risks, you must be aware that accidents can happen and seek to avoid them.

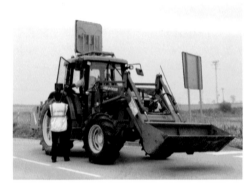

Why do accidents at work occur?

Accidents are not matters of chance. To think that accidents are due to chance is a grave mistake; this would mean that all promotion of safety at work is useless and that we should accept that they are inevitable. In fact, it is common knowledge that accidents at work can be avoided.

Basic causes and immediate causes

Root causes should not be confused with immediate causes. For example, the immediate cause of an accident might be the lack of protective clothing, but the root cause could be that the protective clothing was not used because it was uncomfortable. Thus, when a worker gets a wood or metal shaving in his eye and the incident is investigated, it is often found that he was not wearing his safety glasses. The immediate cause is the absence of individual protection, but the root cause needs to be established and it is crucial to investigate why he was not wearing his glasses. It could have been because it was not specified in that job that you had to use glasses (a lack of working rules), or because the glasses were uncomfortable, etc. It is therefore essential to find out and eliminate the root causes of accidents, because if you only take action on the immediate causes, accidents will surely continue to occur.

Root causes

Root causes can be divided into personal factors and work factors. The most common of these are:

Personal factors:
- Lack of knowledge or capacity to do the work required.
- Lack of motivation or wrong motivation.
- Trying to save time or effort and/or avoiding inconvenience.
- Getting the attention of others, expressing hostility.

Unsafe conditions

- Lack of protection and security in machinery and installations.

- Inadequate protection and security.

- Lack of a warning system, an alarm, or a means of alert.

- Lack of order and cleanliness in the workplace.

- Scarcity of space for working and storing materials.

- Incorrect storage of materials, disorderly stacking, items left in the walkways, piles of material obstructing emergency exits, etc.

- Excessive noise levels.

- Inadequate illumination (lack of light, illuminating lamps, etc.).

- Failure to indicate danger zones.

- Existence of combustible and inflammable materials close to heat sources.

- Existence of unprotected cavities, wells, and ditches that are not indicated and are at risk of causing falls.

- Floors in a poor state; uneven, slippery, and breaking up.

- Lack of railings and other protection on platforms and scaffolding.

- Existence of physical or mental problems or deficiencies.

Work factors:
- Lack of working procedures or unsuitable working procedures.
- Unsuitable design or maintenance of machinery and related equipment.
- Incorrect working practices.
- Normal usage and wear of equipment and tools.
- Abnormal and incorrect use of equipment, tools, and installations.

Immediate causes
Immediate causes can be divided into unsafe actions and unsafe conditions

Unsafe actions are:
- Work being done by those who are not properly qualified.
- Working in unsafe conditions or working too quickly.
- Not giving warning or indicating dangerous conditions that are present.
- Not using, or bypassing, the safety mechanisms with which machinery or installations are equipped.
- Using tools or equipment that are faulty, or in a poor state.
- Not using prescribed individual protective clothing or using unsuitable clothing.
- Playing practical jokes at work.
- Inadequate repair of machinery or installations.
- Repairs carried out by those who are unqualified.

- Adopting incorrect postures when working, especially when manhandling loads.
- Using unsuitable working clothes (with belts or bits hanging off them or torn, or too loose and stained with grease, etc.).
- Wearing rings, bracelets, necklaces, and medals, etc., when working on machinery with moving parts (risk of entanglement).
- Using cables, chains, ropes, slings, and lifting equipment in a poor state of repair.

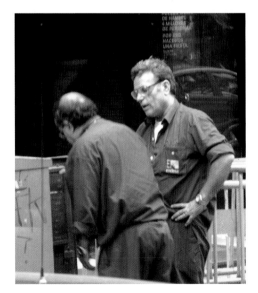

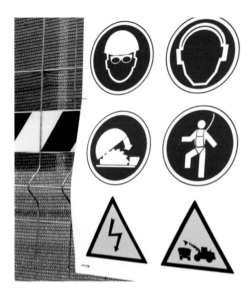

• Exceeding the load capacity of lifting equipment or industrial vehicles.

• Standing beneath suspended loads.

• Getting into ditches, vats, or enclosed spaces without taking due precautions.

• Transporting people on industrial vehicles or carts.

How are injuries caused?

The breaking of a rope or cable securing a load, the collapse of some scaffolding, and a tractor overturning, etc., are accidents, even if nobody is injured. Injuries and accidents are the result of unsafe actions and/or technical failures.

Human error

The reasons why unsafe actions are committed can be classified under the category of human error. Such reasons may be:

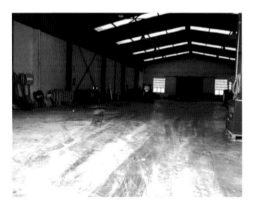

• Physical or mental problems in performing the work correctly; insufficient strength, sight or hearing impairment, excessive nervousness, slow reflexes, and poor understanding, etc.

• Lack of instruction for performing specific tasks.

• Imprudence, negligence, or an obstructive attitude, etc.

Normally the reason for human error lies outside the working environment. It is due to factors associated with what is known as the "social environment."

Focus of prevention

Risk prevention at work may be classified under the following headings:

• **Safety at work.** This is based on the study and analysis of the risks in different workplaces, in order to eliminate or reduce them to tolerable limits, so as to achieve a steady reduction in accidents.

Unsafe actions and technical failures

People ought to be extremely vigilant about keeping to safety regulations where machinery is concerned.

• **Industrial hygiene.** This consists of the recognition, evaluation, and control of those chemical, physical, and biological aspects of the workplace environment which can give rise to illness, destroy health and welfare, or create significant discomfort among workers.

• **Ergonomics.** This has the aim of improving man's adjustment to the technological means of production and to his working and living environment.

Applied psychosociology. The basic objective is to reduce unsafe behavior and imprudent conduct, which are among the most frequent causes of accidents at work.

• **Health awareness.** Among other things, this involves regular medical examinations of workers, their training and supervision regarding

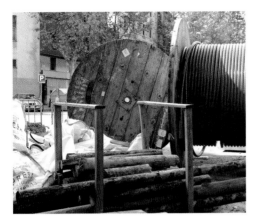

mutual assistance and first aid, or the documenting and filing of personal medical information.

• **Worker training.** Sufficient and suitable training achieves an improved capability and ensures that staff behave in a more safety-conscious manner.

Reducing risk at work

Working accidents and injuries represent one of the principal causes of death and disability. In order to reduce these risks to a minimum, you should:

• Always follow safety instructions.
• Wear suitable protective clothing.
• Use ear protectors or earplugs if you work in a noisy environment.
• Speak to the relevant supervisor if you have any doubts about safety.
• Never drink alcohol during working hours.

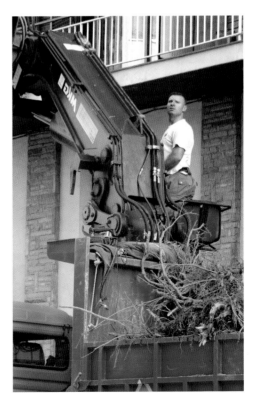

Despite the fact that safety and hygiene measures have improved in the working environment over recent years, there are still many people who have accidents, or develop work-related illnesses. To reduce this, it is essential to ascertain the number of injuries and illnesses and how they are caused and to scrupulously respect various basic norms of behavior.

As many as 79.3 percent of workers have physical ailments that may be related to their working postures and workload.

The mental pressure to which workers are subjected is even greater. Thus, the high degree of concentration required, the accelerated pace of work, or the amount of tasks performed, are factors that take a psychological toll on workers. The symptoms developed by them due to such work pressures tend to be alterations in sleep patterns, tiredness, headaches, lack of concentration, and irritability, etc.

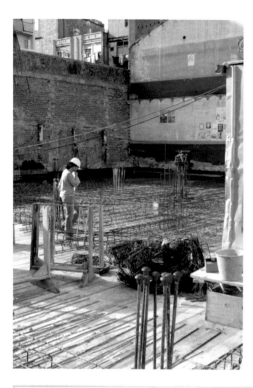
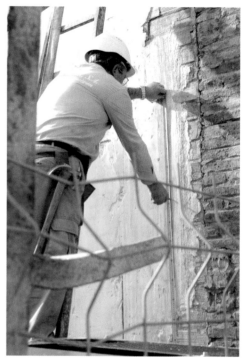

Advice

- Work the proper hours: doing overtime or an excessive working day causes a greater number of accidents and injuries.

- Walkways and exits should remain free of obstacles.

- The workplace should be clean and orderly.

- If you handle loads, keep your back straight and your feet firmly supported.

- If there is any electrical fault, it is best to inform the maintenance team, instead of trying to solve the problem yourself.

- Do not connect different electrical appliances to the same socket.

- If you handle chemical products at work, you must use suitable protection and be aware of the phone number to use in an emergency.

- If you spend your working day in front of a monitor, your back should be straight and your seat adjusted to the right height. There should be no reflections from the screen. The minimum distance of your eyes from the computer or television should be 16 inches (40 cm) and you should change position after every two hours of work.

- Professionals who use a vehicle for their work should respect road safety rules and wear a safety belt.

- Stress can be avoided or reduced if tasks are suitably planned, with the heaviest workload at the beginning of the day and by taking rest breaks.

- The manager should keep the workplace in a proper condition: electrical installations, heating, extinguishers, or sprinklers should be checked regularly and updated to promote safety in the working environment.

- Finally, it is advisable to carry out routine medical examinations as established by the company's health and safety department. If a worker is self-employed, he should check his health regularly; it is the best way of preventing illness or dealing with health complications in time.

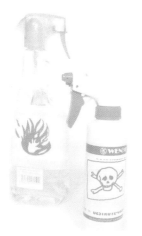

Cleaning products

Among cleaning products are some that, by their nature, represent a serious risk for consumers and workers who use them habitually and they should thus be considered dangerous substances. However, if some minimal precautions are adopted, these products can be used without any risk whatsoever.

Cleaning products

For your health and safety, before using such products, you must be aware of their characteristics, which are stated on their containers and labels, in accordance with legal requirements.

Commonly used products should not include any that are potentially carcinogenic, mutagenic, or have toxic effects on the reproductive system.

A household product is defined as a substance used for household maintenance and cleaning or for the personal care of its users. The use of such products is the third most common cause of severe poisoning, after alcohol and drugs, amounting to 15–30 percent of all registered cases.

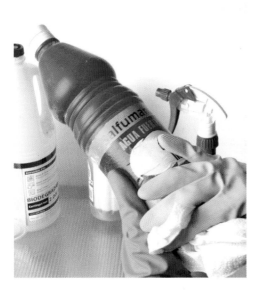

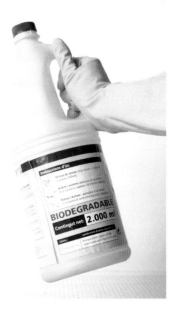

Classification of dangerous substances

Any preparation qualifies as being dangerous if it has the capacity to harm people, property, or the environment, directly or indirectly.

Substances can be categorized according to the different dangers they pose, depending on their chemical and physical properties:

• **Explosive:** when they can explode as a result of fire or are sensitive to movement and shocks.

• **Oxidizing:** substances that cause combustion, incandescence, or flames, or which can cause them to happen.

• **Extremely flammable:** products that burn easily and catch fire immediately.

• **Highly flammable:**

– Substances or preparations that may heat up or catch fire in the air at atmospheric temperature without any external contribution of energy.

Some preparations contain more than one dangerous substance, so the harmful effects are potentially worse.

– Solids that can catch fire easily through brief contact with a heat source and that continue burning or being consumed after the heat source has been removed.

– Liquids with a very low point of ignition.

– When in contact with water or moist air, easily flammable gases are given off in dangerous quantities.

• **Flammable:** capable of catching fire immediately.

• **Very toxic:** highly poisonous.

• **Toxic:** capable of causing severe risks to health, however they are absorbed.

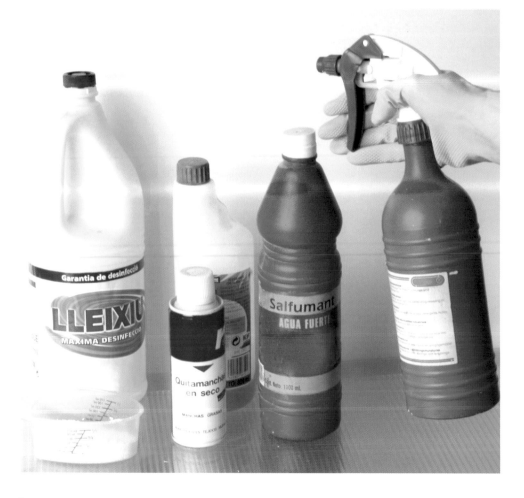

SYMBOLS AND INDICATIONS OF HAZARD FOR DANGEROUS SUBSTANCES AND PREPARATIONS

Meaning	Symbol	Description of risks	Examples of products	Preventive measures
Dangerous for the environment (N)		- Substances very toxic for aquatic organisms. - Toxic for wildlife. - Dangerous for the ozone layer.	- Active substances in pesticides. - Chlorofluorocarbons (CFCs).	- Eliminate the product or its remains as dangerous waste. - Avoid contamination of the environment by means of appropriate storage.
Toxic (T) Very toxic (T+) Harmful (Xn)		- Toxic and harmful substances and preparations that, even in small quantities, are a health hazard. - If they have serious effects on health, even in very small quantities, the product is indicated by a toxicity symbol. - These products enter the body by inhalation, ingestion or through the skin.	- Methanol, alcohol for burning, stain removers, - Disinfectants, - Paints, - Stain removers, solvents like trichloroethylene, painting solvents, and cleaning products. - Products for protecting and treating wood. - Paint strippers.	- To avoid all contact with the skin, use a means of protection: gloves, a screen. and overalls, etc. - Preferably work outside or in a well-ventilated place. - Suitable hygiene: wash your hands and never eat or smoke during use. - Aerosol products are more dangerous (inhalation). Keep away from children when using them. - Keep these products out of children's reach.
Corrosive (C)		- Corrosive substances seriously damage living tissue and also attack other materials. The reaction can be due to the presence of water or humidity.	- Pipe unblocking products, descalers. - Caustic soda. - Acids, sulfuric acid. - Oven and sink cleaners. - Dishwasher products (in a wet state).	- Keep the products in their original container (well closed and with safety instructions). - Keep these products out of children's reach. - Be careful where you put them, never leave them on window ledges, etc. (risk of falling). - Protect your eyes and skin, etc., against splashes. Be very careful when pouring or spraying the product. - Always use protective gloves and eyeglasses. - Hygiene is vital: after use, wash your face and hands well. - For first aid, washing it out with a lot of water for ten minutes is effective. - Corrosive products in aerosols are dangerous.

Explosive (E)		An explosion is an extremely rapid combustion, which depends on the characteristics of the product, on temperature (heat source), on contact with other products (reaction), on shocks and movement, etc.	All types of aerosols, including empty ones, are potential bombs above 122 °F (50°C): air purifiers, hairsprays, paints, varnishes and deicers for windshields, etc.	- Avoid excessive heat and knocks, protect it from the sun's rays. - Never place it near heat sources, lamps and radiators, etc.
Irritant (Xi)		- Repeated contact with irritant products causes inflammatory reactions in the skin and mucus membranes.	- Bleach. - Turpentine substitute. - Ammonia. - Polyester putty.	The same as for Toxic products
Highly inflammable (F) Extremely inflammable (F+)		- (F) Highly inflammable products burn in contact with a flame, a heat source (hot surface) or a spark. - (F+) Products that can catch fire very easily, reacting to an energy source (flame and spark, etc.), even below 32°F (0°C).	- Petroleum, gasoline. - Burning alcohol or methanol. - Turpentine substitute. - Mineral turpentine. - Acetone, paintbrush cleaners, paint solvents. - Aerosol paints, metallic paints. - Deicers. - Contact glues, glues (neoprene). - Air purifiers.	- Store these products in a well-ventilated place. - Never use them near a heat source, a hot surface, sparks or an unprotected flame. - Never smoke! - Do not wear nylon clothing and always have an extinguisher within reach when using these flammable products. - Keep these flammable products (F) well away from oxidizing products (O).
Oxidizing (O)		- Combustion requires a combustible material, oxygen, and a flammable source: the reaction accelerates considerably in the presence of an oxidizing product (a substance rich in oxygen).	The same as for Flammable products	The same as for Flammable products

MOUTH-TO-MOUTH RESUSCITATION		
Adults	**Children**	**Babies**
1 breath every five seconds	1 breath every three seconds	1 breath every three seconds
12 breaths/minute	20 breaths/minute	30–40 breaths/minute

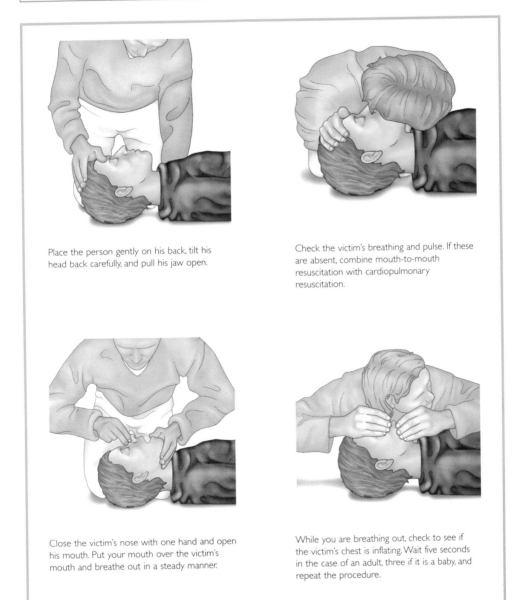

Place the person gently on his back, tilt his head back carefully, and pull his jaw open.

Check the victim's breathing and pulse. If these are absent, combine mouth-to-mouth resuscitation with cardiopulmonary resuscitation.

Close the victim's nose with one hand and open his mouth. Put your mouth over the victim's mouth and breathe out in a steady manner.

While you are breathing out, check to see if the victim's chest is inflating. Wait five seconds in the case of an adult, three if it is a baby, and repeat the procedure.

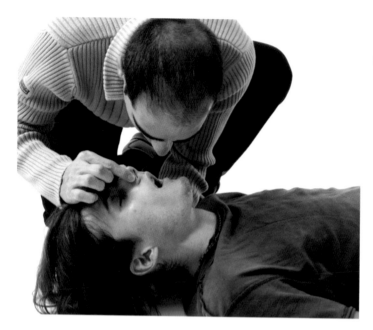

Place the person gently on his back, tilting his head back carefully, and open his jaw. Block the victim's nose with one hand and open his mouth. Put your mouth over the victim's mouth and breathe out steadily. While you are breathing out, check if the victim's chest is inflating. Wait 5 seconds if it is an adult, 3 if it is a baby, and repeat the procedure.

tion and breathing will not be affected by anything that may constrict.

• Remove any foreign bodies from the victim's mouth.

• If you have verified that the victim has no pulse, you must combine mouth-to-mouth resuscitation with cardiopulmonary resuscitation.

• This technique must be performed until medical assistance arrives, since it is very important to maintain the supply of oxygen to the victim's brain.

Cardiopulmonary resuscitation

• Cardiopulmonary resuscitation is performed when the victim has no pulse and is not breathing.

• It consists of combining mouth-to-mouth resuscitation with cardiac massage.

• With this technique, you can keep the lungs full of oxygen and try to make the blood circulate, ensuring that it reaches the brain and other parts of the body.

What is the pulse

The pulse is the rhythmic force produced by the heart with every beat and is perceptible in any artery near the surface of the body, such as the temples, wrists, the inside of the arm, or the groin.

Method

• Check if the victim is breathing and has a pulse. If not:

• Place the victim on his back with his legs stretched out and his arms next to his body. Lift his chin while moving his forehead backward.

• Place the palms of your hands one on top of the other, with the fingers stretched out above the sternum, as shown in the picture.

• If the victim is a child, only use one hand. If he is a baby, use only the index and middle fingers, placing them in the middle of his chest.

The pupil reflex

• The pupil reflex is used to rule out brain injuries or signs of other illness.

• How to induce the pupil reflex:

– Shine a small flashlight into the eye and see if the pupil contracts.

– If a flashlight is unavailable, open the eye suddenly by lifting the upper eyelid and see if the pupil contracts.

• If the pupils seem larger than normal, it can be a sign of hemorrhaging, heatstroke, or that substances like cocaine or amphetamines have been taken.

• If the pupils are smaller than normal, it can be a sign of sunstroke or the use of sleeping drugs.

• If, when shining a light at the pupils, one pupil does not contract, or they are not the

CHEST COMPRESSION				
	Adults		**Children**	
1 person assisting	15 chest compressions every two breaths	80/100 compressions per minute	5 chest compressions every breath	80/100 compressions per minute
2 people assisting	5 chest compressions every breath and change position	80/100 compressions per minute	Cannot be done	Cannot be done

The position that is adopted while performing chest compressions on the accident victim

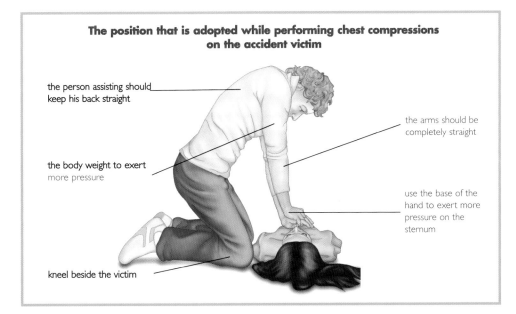

the person assisting should keep his back straight

the arms should be completely straight

the body weight to exert more pressure

use the base of the hand to exert more pressure on the sternum

kneel beside the victim

same size, head injuries or paralysis may be suspected.

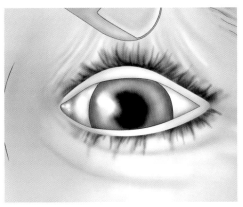

A medical flashlight being shone into an eye.

Important

The cardiopulmonary resuscitation procedure should be stopped when the victim's pulse and breathing return.

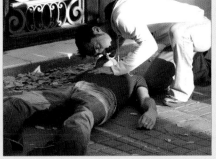

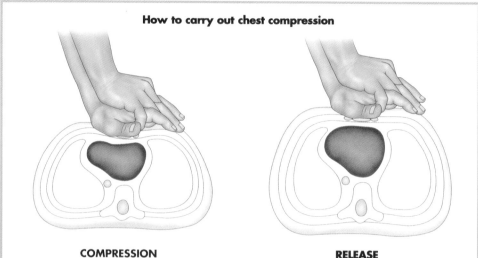

How to carry out chest compression

COMPRESSION

Compress the chest gently and leave your hands on the victim's chest. By compressing the sternum by 1.5 to 2 inches (4 to 5 cm) , you can help the heart to expel blood.

RELEASE

When the pressure on the sternum is released, the elasticity of the chest wall makes the heart and the chest expand and fill with blood (thoracic diastole); in the process, the blood is oxygenated in the lungs.

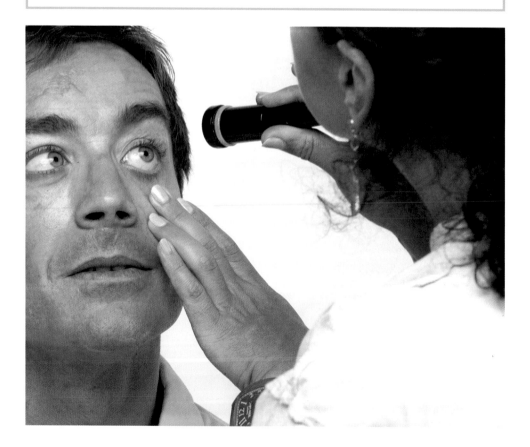

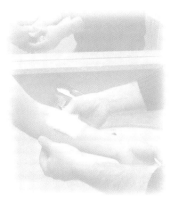

Wounds and bleeding

Immediate intervention is vital in certain emergency situations that occur in daily life. For this reason, it is a great help to have a basic idea of first aid that allows you to treat minor wounds and even to be able to apply a tourniquet in the case of a more severe hemorrhage, before requesting medical assistance, if necessary.

If the wound is minor

The procedure for wounds is based on controlling their immediate consequences (bleeding, internal injuries), preventing subsequent complications through contamination (infection), and aiding the healing process. Thus, the steps to be followed are:

• Whoever is assisting should remain calm and keep the victim calm too. Tell him at each

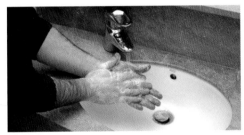

1. Wash your hands with soap and water. Wash all the instruments you are going to use with alcohol: scissors and tweezers, etc.

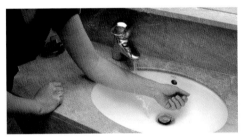

2. Wash the wound under a faucet with soap and water, gently and without rubbing, so as to remove possible foreign bodies.

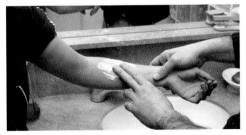

3. Apply an antiseptic solution or iodine.

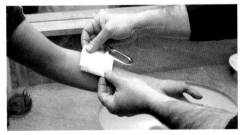

4. Use sterile gauze to finish cleaning the wound. Always do this from the inside to the outside of the wound. Moving the gauze in this way prevents germs entering the wound. The sterile gauze must not be reused.

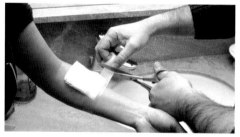

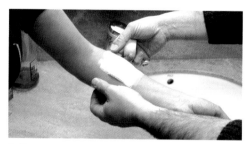

5. If any hairs or pieces of skin have been left hanging, cut them away gently with blunt-ended scissors.

6. Place a sterile dressing over the wound to keep it free of germs and accelerate the healing process. Secure the dressing with adhesive dressing tape.

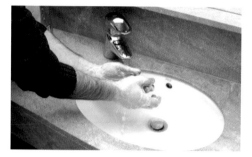

7. Repeat this procedure every day to keep the wound clean.

moment the procedures you are going to carry out.

If the wound is serious

With minor bleeding, you should concentrate on stopping the loss of blood. If it is serious, you must also administer liquids. The steps to follow are:

• Whoever is treating the wound should remain calm and keep the injured person calm, too. The victim should be told at each moment what procedure is going to be performed.

• Control the bleeding by pressing on the points shown in the illustration.

• If the wound has foreign bodies inside it, do not try to remove them, because of the danger of exacerbating the wound.

• Also, do not poke around inside the wound.

• Place a sterile gauze over it.

• If the gauze gets soaked in blood, put a new one over it, without taking off the first one.

• Put a bandage over the wound:

– Take the victim to the emergency room.

– In the meantime, keep the injured limb raised up (above the level of the heart).

General advice

• A tourniquet should always be positioned between the wound and the heart. Bandages or

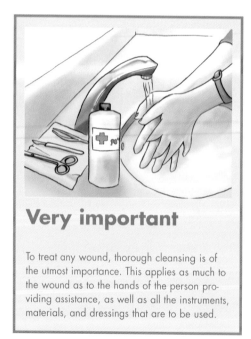

Very important

To treat any wound, thorough cleansing is of the utmost importance. This applies as much to the wound as to the hands of the person providing assistance, as well as all the instruments, materials, and dressings that are to be used.

▪ What not to do

• Cleaning the wound with alcohol, since this can cause burns around it.

• Cleaning the wound with cotton swabs, because this can leave threads inside the wound and delay healing.

soft fabrics should be used, which are as wide as possible. These bandages should be at least 4 inches (10 cm) wide.

• Place gauze to act as a cushion over the wound. Pass the bandage that will be used for the tourniquet twice over the wound and make a half-knot.

• Place a long object, like a pencil or stick, over the half-knot that has been made and complete the tourniquet.

• Twist the pencil or stick until you see that the bleeding has stopped. At this point, do not twist any more or exert more pressure.

• The tourniquet should remain visible at all times and not be covered with clothing or blankets.

• Write a note on the bandage, clearly indicating the time when the tourniquet was applied.

• Loosen the tourniquet every 20 minutes to allow the blood to circulate, but never remove it. The total period during which the tourniquet remains applied should never exceed two hours. If the tourniquet is left on longer than necessary, it can cause gangrene in the limb, which would then have to be amputated.

• Cover the accident victim with a blanket (but leaving the tourniquet visible), since hemorrhaging causes body temperature to fall.

Hemorrhages in specific areas

The face and skull

• Cover the area with a gauze or clean dressing.
• If no fracture is suspected, exert direct pressure until the bleeding stops.

The nose

(epistaxis or nose bleeding)
• Make the victim sit down. The sitting position reduces the supply of blood to the head and nose.
• If necessary, lean the head forward to avoid blood being swallowed, which could cause vomiting.
• Press on the sides of the nose (above the nostrils) with your index finger and thumb. This obstructs the main artery that supplies blood to the nose.
• If bleeding continues, plug the nose with gauze moistened with distilled or boiled water.

Bandaging a wound, step by step

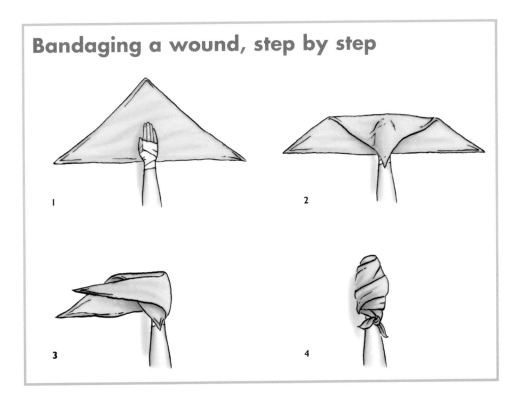

1

2

3

4

When to make a tourniquet

A tourniquet is a bandage that exerts pressure on the arteries around the wound. Its function is to stop the hemorrhage. It is a very dangerous procedure, which must only be performed in the following cases:

- When you have tried to stop the hemorrhaging by other means and failed. Before considering the possibility of making a tourniquet, you should try to stop the bleeding by exerting strong pressure upon the wound, or upon the arterial pressure points mentioned below, or by raising up the injured limb.

- If a limb has been completely severed. Normally, in this case, bleeding does not begin immediately, but it can commence at any moment, which is why a tourniquet may be left on to exert pressure on the wound when necessary.

- If the bleeding is so intense that it endangers the victim's life.

- A tourniquet, once applied and tightened up, should never be removed except by trained medical personnel, because removing it without due medical precautions would aggravate the state of shock, possibly even causing the sudden death of the victim.

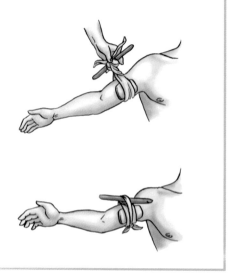

- Apply cold water compresses or ice (wrapped in a gauze towel or compress) over the forehead and the nose.
- Do not expose to the sun.
- Do not allow the patient to sleep, because this increases the bleeding.
- Take him to a medical center.

Inside the mouth
(alveolar hemorrhage)
- Plug the alveolus—the hole in the gum that is bleeding—with gauze soaked in oxygenated water (diluted) and tell the patient to bite strongly.
- Do not allow him to rinse it with any kind of solution and especially not with lukewarm water.
- Do not give him any alcoholic drinks.
- Do not allow anything to enter the alveolus, such as ash, salt, coffee, etc.
- Take him for an examination by a doctor.

Female genital hemorrhage
- Make the patient lie down in a horizontal posi-

tion and reassure her. Cover her up to prevent her getting cold.
- If sanitary towels are not available, use dressings or gauze.
- Constantly monitor her breathing and pulse.
- If she is conscious, give her sweet drinks.
- Do not give her any alcoholic drinks.
- Take her immediately to the emergency room, keeping her in a horizontal position.

Signs of an internal hemorrhage
Very sensitive or rigid abdomen, hematomas (red patches caused by bleeding under the skin) on different parts of the body.
- Loss of blood from the rectum or vagina.
- Vomiting with blood.
- Simple fractures.
- Signs of shock.

Dealing with internal hemorrhages
- If the victim has symptoms of internal hemor-

Arterial compression

When the arterial wound is located in the neck, armpit, or groin, a tourniquet is contraindicated, so you should therefore exert manual compression until medical assistance arrives.

Method of arterial compression

1. Carotid. Compression is applied by the thumb on the carotid artery with the rest of the hand on the back of the neck.

Subclavian. Compression is applied by the thumb on the subclavian artery with the rest of the hand on the back of the shoulder.

2. Armpit. Compression is applied by the thumb on the wound with the rest of the hand behind the armpit, without lifting the arm.

3. Humeral. Compression is applied by the thumb on the wound with the rest of the hand on the back of the arm, with the arm slightly raised.

4. Femoral. Compression is applied by the fist placed along the artery

The arterial compression method is a method that proves effective in some specific cases. It should only be used if the treatments described earlier are impossible or inappropriate, since its use has some disadvantages:

- It requires a good knowledge of anatomy.
- It cannot be maintained for a long time because the person applying it gets exhausted.
- It requires the continued presence of a person with one accident victim, when they might be needed to assist another.

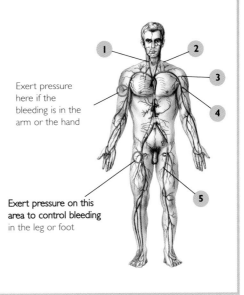

Exert pressure here if the bleeding is in the arm or the hand

Exert pressure on this area to control bleeding in the leg or foot

---

rhaging, or you suspect that the force of the injury was sufficient to cause this, take the victim as soon as possible to hospital.

- Check breathing and pulse every 5 minutes.
- Cover the victim up.
- Do not give the victim anything to eat or drink.

▪ Internal hemorrhage

An internal hemorrhage is one where the blood does not flow to the outside of the body, but remains inside, generally accumulating under the skin or in an organ cavity, the latter case being more severe. Internal hemorrhages include serious injuries that may cause shock, heart attacks, or lung failure. They can be caused by crushing, puncturing, ruptures in organs and blood vessels, and by fractures. All types of hemorrhage cause a reduction in the supply of blood circulating, which the body tries to conserve, especially in the most important organs, such as: the heart, brain, and lungs.

271

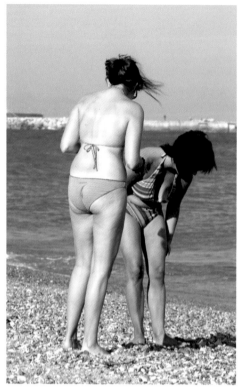

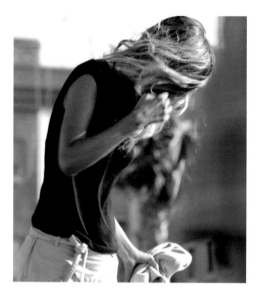

It is essential to have a first aid kit at home, at work, in the car, or anywhere that people gather. This should have the materials that are indispensable for attending to casualties when you have minimal knowledge or none at all. The first aid kit is often of decisive importance in certain situations. Its contents may vary according to where it is located.

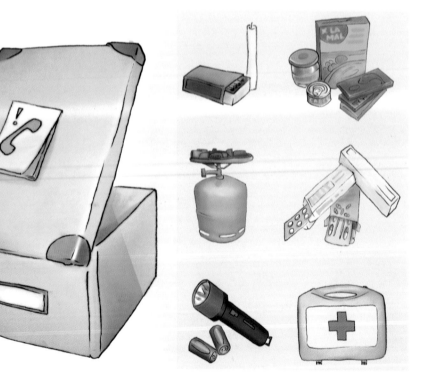

Bandages

Putting on a bandage is not at all difficult if you are used to doing it, but for someone who is not familiar with this procedure, it can be a problem. Other techniques, such as making a sling, can be very useful in arm injuries and easy to perform. If you are not sure how to do it, it is better to leave this to a professional.

General considerations regarding bandages

• During bandaging, the victim should be placed in a comfortable position, bearing in mind also the comfort of the person who is going to put on the bandage, since some types of bandage need time to put on.

• Choose bandages the right size for the area you are going to bandage.

• The bandage always should begin from the part of the limb that is furthest from the body. Thus, for example, if you are going to bandage an arm, you should begin from the wrist in the direction of the shoulder, and in the case of a leg, you should begin from the ankle in the direction of the thigh. The reason for bandaging in this direction is to avoid blood accumulation in the furthest part of the limb.

• Bandaging is normally done from left to right.

• When winding the bandage around for the first time, angle it at 45° toward the body, and the second time, at 45° in the opposite direction to the first loop, that is to say, away from the body. The third loop should be like the first and so on, alternating, until the bandage has a spiral or criss-cross appearance.

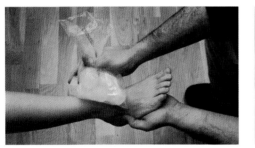

1

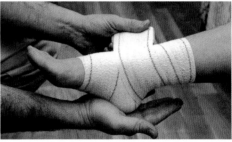

2

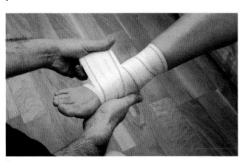

3

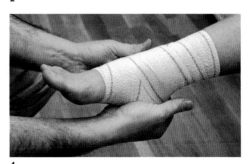

4

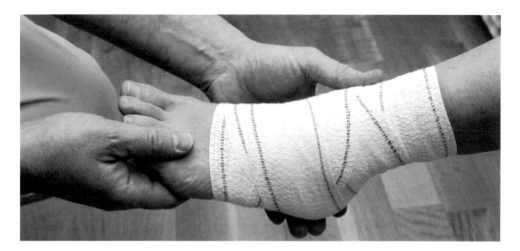

Always bandage in the direction of the heart to avoid the accumulation of blood in the furthest part of the limb that is being immobilized.

• Unroll the bandage as required, not excessively, to avoid bandages that are too loose or too tight. The pressure applied should be uniform for the whole bandaging procedure, to avoid excessive pressure on some areas with others looser than the rest.

• If the victim gets a prickling sensation in the area, or his skin changes color, or the area feels cold, take off the bandage and begin again.

• The bandage should finish in an area away from the injury. The end of the bandage should be secured with adhesive tape or safety pins.

• Do not use more bandaging than necessary. If there is too much, trim it with scissors and secure it appropriately.

Types of bandages

How to bandage an ankle

• Begin by putting two strips of bandage on the leg, below the inside and outside ankle bones, and finish off in the front area of the leg, always being careful not to bandage too tightly, in case you inhibit blood circulation in the leg.

• Put on a third strip of bandage, this time under the big and little toes of the foot.

• This third strip of bandage should be put on in a U-shape. Secure it to the first bandage that was put on, passing it under the heel.

• This last U-shaped bandage should be fixed to the ankle. It should be attached appropriately,

exerting a little pressure with your fingers, taking care not to damage the ankle.

• Put on a C-shaped strip around the Achilles' tendon and take it toward the strip that goes round the big and little toes of the foot. Then, attach it here.

• Repeat the bandage in figure 3, but this time, shifting the position of the bandaging slightly more forward.

• Then repeat the bandage in figure 4. The procedure shown in the last two figures is repeated, until three U-shaped bandages and three C-shaped bandages have been completed.

• Put on another strip of bandage, which goes from the outside of the ankle to the inside of the heel. The part of the bandage that goes over the outside of the ankle will cover the one from the inside of the heel. This bandage will be fixed to the first piece of bandaging, as shown in figure 1. Repeat the procedure, but in reverse, starting the bandage from the inside of the ankle and finishing at the outside of the heel.

• Put on bandages like those in figure 1, but moved slightly downward to stabilize those that have just been fixed to it.

• Repeat the procedure, shifting each strip of bandage a little further downward, until reaching the instep of the foot.

• Put on another bandage to secure those that have just been attached.

• Make sure all the bandages remain well secured.

How to make a sling with a triangular bandage

• To make a triangular bandage, use a rectangular sheet or article of clothing that is no longer required. Cut it with scissors into a triangle with a base of 5 feet (1.5 m) and whose sides are both 3 feet (90 cm) in length.

• If no scissors are available, you can take a rectangular piece of material and fold it diagonally into the shape of a triangle.

• If the sling is for a child, cut off a smaller area, to fit his size.

• The piece of fabric is hung over the opposite shoulder to the injury and is passed under the injured arm. The upper point of the triangle you have made should be at the elbow on the injured arm.

• Tie the two free ends of the cloth triangle behind the victim's neck. This step should be done carefully so that the arm is at the correct height and is bent in a comfortable position.

• If you want to immobilize the injured arm even more, use another piece of cloth and tie it around the body. Slings should not be either very tight or very loose, to ensure that the limb has suitable blood circulation.

How to bandage a hand

• Wind the bandage around twice at the wrist.

Take the bandage toward the fingers and wind it around twice in a circular fashion and twice passing below the thumb.

• Pass the bandage again between the thumb and the wrist.

• Finish with a couple of loops around the wrist and tie it up.

How to make a triangular sling

1. Cut out a triangle from a piece of fabric that is 5 feet (1.5 meters) wide.

2. Another way could be to fold double a large piece of square fabric to make a triangle. If the sling is for a child, the size can be reduced.

3. To put on the sling, place the victim's elbow in the upper point of the triangle and his wrist halfway along the bottom side opposite it. Then tie the two free ends of the triangle to the shoulder on the same side, or on the opposite shoulder. The height of the knot should be adjusted in such a way that the elbow remains bent at the correct angle.

4. If there is no material to cut a triangle out of, cut up a coat or undershirt. Then fix the sling in the way shown in the illustration. You can also make slings with belts, ropes, strong netting, or sheets.

5. If it is necessary to immobilize the injured arm, attach the sling to the body with another piece of cloth, around the chest, and tie it up on the healthy side.

6. It is important to check periodically that the sling is not too tight; if so, loosen it.

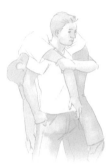

Injured people

Transporting accident victims should always be done in a very careful manner, since abrupt movements while they are being carried or eventual falls can worsen the state of the casualty. It is always best for this to be done by two or more people to spread the weight of the victim suitably.

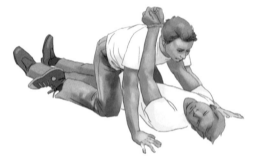

General advice

• It is not advisable to transport a casualty until the emergency medical services have arrived; they will be responsible for dealing with the victim's injuries appropriately. Only in extreme cases, such as floods, fires, danger of electrocution, or asphyxia, should you move the casualty, because you run the risk of aggravating his state of health.

• As a general rule, it is best to move the victim as though he were a single immobile block.

• If there is a chair available, use it.

• If you have belts or straps at your disposal, these can be used, too.

• Always when moving a casualty, you must check the position of the victim's back and neck at every moment, to avoid awkward movements and possible injuries.

• Before lifting an individual, you should calculate his weight and assess whether you can manage it.

• If there are other people at the accident site, it is best to ask for their help.

• While transporting the victim, those people responsible for carrying him should keep their

backs straight. To lift him up and move him, you should use the strength in your legs.

• When you have agreed with the other people about transporting the casualty, decide beforehand where you are going to take him.

• Remember that if several people are carrying him, the person nearest to the victim's head must always have the task of directing the operation.

Dragging the casualty

• This type of rescue should only be used when the casualty is in very urgent need of evacuation and the distance to cover is less than about 10 yards (9 m).

• Only do this when the ground is flat, like the floor of a building. It is not advisable in the mountains or in a place with stairs.

The method to adopt is the following:

– Kneel over the victim, as he lies on his back.

– If the victim is conscious, let him clasp his hands around your neck.

– If the victim is unconscious, tie his hands with an article of clothing around the wrists and put them around your neck.

• If you judge that the victim is too heavy to drag this way, you can pull him by his feet if that is easier, although you should be careful that the casualty does not get bumped over uneven areas of ground.

• If the victim is light or is a child, it is better to carry him on your shoulders:

– Make the casualty kneel down, putting your arms around him under his armpits.

– Lift him up and lean him against a wall.

– Bend down allowing the victim's weight to go

With two people

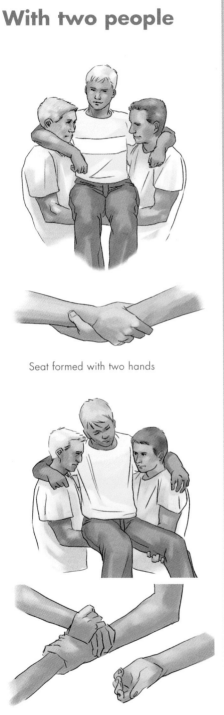

Seat formed with two hands

Seat formed with three hands

The fireman's method

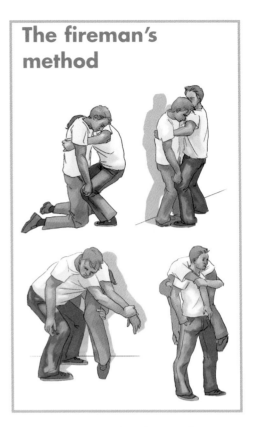

over your shoulder and putting one of your arms between the casualty's thighs.

– Then stand up, holding the victim strongly by one leg and one arm. This position allows you one free arm.

The fireman's method
With two people assisting
Seat formed with two hands
• If this method is adopted, the two people lift the victim from under his thighs, linking their wrists, and the other two arms of the people assisting are used to support the victim's back.
Seat formed with three hands
• A variation of the previous method is the so-called "three-hand chair," in which the two arms of one person pass under the victim's thighs, linking together with one arm of the other person (see picture). The free arm of one person can be used to support one of the victim's legs, if it is injured.

Transporting the victim with a chair
• This method takes advantage of a chair's rigidity.
• To do this, one person gets in front of the chair and the other behind, as shown in the illustration.

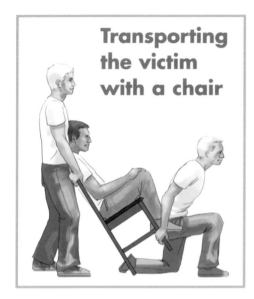

Transporting the victim with a chair

With three people assisting

• The first person places his arms under the victim's anklebones, the second under his buttocks and the third under his neck and back.

• The three have to cooperate and kneel down at the same time, moving the victim as though he were a solid immobile block.

• Finally, the three get up at the same time. The chest of the victim should be facing the people assisting him.

How to move the casualty if a stretcher is available

• The stretcher must be brought to the victim and not vice versa. The stretcher should be placed on the ground and the victim moved as gently as possible, remembering that he should always be treated as a solid immobile block.

• Once the victim has been placed on the stretcher, he should be covered with a blanket, because being immobilized may make him lose body heat more easily.

• If the stretcher has straps, these should be used, since if any of the people assisting fall or if they make any abrupt movements, this could aggravate the victim's injuries.

• The stretcher should be lifted with the greatest of care. Each stretcher-bearer should kneel down at either end of the stretcher and when the bearer at the back gives the word, they should stand up.

• The stretcher should be carried in a horizontal position at all times.

When the victim has no serious injuries

• **Carrying in your arms:** This is a very practical method for moving people who are not too heavy or children (depending on the physique of the person assisting) and who are not seriously injured, with a sprain for example.

– It consists in holding the victim, placing one hand under his knees so as to support his legs and the other around his back, supporting the weight of his trunk; the victim can hold on to the person assisting by putting his arms around his neck.

– You must be particularly careful when lifting the weight of the victim (for example, if he has been sitting on the ground), and make sure you bend your knees when stooping down to avoid making all the effort with your back muscles, which could cause lumbar injuries.

Ways of improvising a stretcher

A stretcher can be improvised in the following manner:

• Get 2 or 3 jackets or coats and 2 strong wooden poles.

• Pull the sleeves of the clothing toward the inside.

• Pass the wooden poles through the sleeves.

• Button up or close the zips of the garments.

Another way of making a stretcher:

• Get a blanket or some canvas and two strong pieces of wood.

• Lay the blanket or the canvas out on the ground.

• Mentally divide the fabric into three parts. Put a piece of wood on the first section and fold the fabric over.

• Place the other piece of wood about 6 inches (15 cm) from the edge of the fabric and fold the fabric over it again.

Rautek maneuver

This is used to remove a casualty from the inside of a car, while protecting his spinal column.

- This maneuver is only carried out by somebody in extreme cases when it is essential to move the victim to save his life: heart and lung failure or a burning vehicle, etc.

- Free the victim's feet if they are trapped by the vehicle's pedals.

- Get close to the victim from one side.

- Slide your arms under the casualty's armpits.

- Hold the victim's arm by the wrist with one hand and, with the other, hold the victim's chin. The injured victim is "leaned" against your chest.

- Move slowly, removing the victim from inside the car and maintaining the head-neck-trunk axis of the victim in the same line, as though these parts of the victim formed a single immobile block.

- When the casualty has been removed, he should be placed with great care and very gradually upon the ground or a stretcher, until medical assistance arrives.

The bridge technique

When you have access to the victim from both sides, this technique can be used to place him on the stretcher.

- The people assisting stand over the victim with their legs apart:

- One holds his head and the upper part of his back.

- The second holds the victim by his hips.

- The third holds his legs under the knees.

- The person situated at the head of the victim gives the order to raise him up.

- A fourth places the stretcher under the victim.

- In unison, the people assisting place the victim on the stretcher.

• **Carrying the casualty on your shoulders or back:** The instructions for this are the same as in the previous method; nevertheless, it does not require as much strength, because the weight of the victim is partly transferred to your trunk. By clasping your hands together, it is easier

How to move a casualty with three people assisting

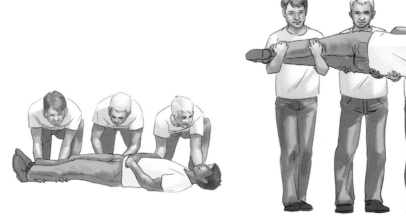

to bear the weight of the victim. This method is of no use for unconscious victims, since it requires the cooperation of the casualty, putting his arms around your neck.

• **With the casualty supporting himself on your shoulder:** A casualty who has no serious injuries and can walk by himself, can be assisted if he puts one of his arms around your neck and his free arm around your waist for additional support. This method can be performed by two people, depending on the size of the victim and the amount of space available, etc. With the help of a third person, supporting the victim's legs, it is possible to go downstairs.

How to move a casualty with five people

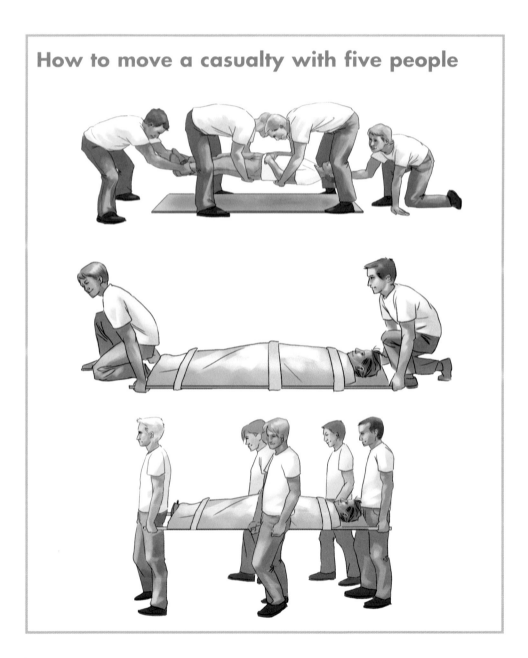

What to do in the case of an earthquake

Earthquakes or seismic events are caused by tremors and abrupt movements of the earth. When an earthquake happens in the sea, it may cause a tsunami or tidal wave. The areas that are close to points of movement between plates of the earth's crust are more prone to this type of natural phenomenon.

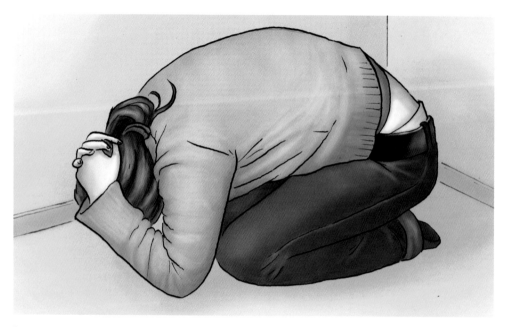

This is one of the most recommended positions in case of an earthquake. Crouch down while making sure that you are not near a shelf or mobile object that might fall on you. Cover your head with your hands and put your head against your knees to protect it.

What to do during an earthquake

• Keep your family calm and also the other people nearby. If you have developed a plan of action for earthquakes as a preventive measure, this should be put into practice.

• Go to the safest place in the house, which should have been located previously and which your family will have been told about. Crouch down and cover your head with your hands, placing your head against your knees.

• Under no circumstances use the elevators.

• Keep away from shelves and mobile household objects.

• Do not get out in a hurry. The majority of earthquakes only last a few seconds and it will probably have finished before you manage to get out of the building.

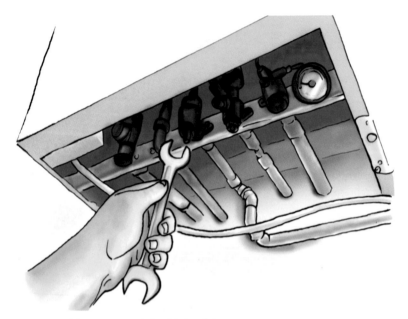

Carefully check all the water, gas, and electricity installations.

• Shut off the electricity supply, the gas, and water, and do not produce any naked flames.

After the earthquake

• Check if there are any injured people, fires, or leaks of toxic substances. If there are, call the emergency services immediately.

• Only use the emergency number in case of serious accidents, to avoid jamming the phone lines. It is best to switch on the radio and listen to the advice of the emergency services.

• In the event of being evacuated from your building by the emergency services, do this calmly without spreading panic to other people and always follow instructions given.

• Do not light matches or lighters until you are sure that the earthquake has not caused any gas leaks.

• Carefully check all the damage caused by the quake to your dwelling. If the cracks are substantial, leave your home and call the emergency services.

• Clean up the house, paying special attention to toxic products, like bleach or ammonia.

• Be alert to aftershocks, which usually occur several minutes after the main earthquake. They are normally of a weaker intensity, but can also cause significant damage.

• If there is food and drink that could have been in contact with toxic substances during the quake, dispose of them immediately, because they will no longer be suitable for consumption.

• If you have been trapped in the rubble, keep calm and wait for the emergency services to arrive. Meanwhile, bang away with some object so that they can hear you.

• The strongest structures inside a building are a load-bearing wall, a pillar, or the corners of rooms. You can also seek protection under solid furniture, like tables or beds.

• If you find yourself outside during an earthquake, it is better to stay in the street and keep away from cornices, windows, and telephone poles.

Being prepared for an earthquake

• Much of the damage caused by earthquakes can be mitigated if you have a basic awareness of the effects of these natural disasters:

• Ensure that pictures, shelves, and potentially dangerous furniture are suitably secured and will therefore not fall over easily in an earthquake.

• Check the electricity, water, and gas installations regularly and monitor the situation inside the house. This information should be shared with the rest of your family.

What to do in the case of heavy winds or storms

Natural disasters, such as floods, very violent storms, and tornados, can seriously endanger the public, and create many problems for local services. If you make even minimal preparations to be able to hold out until the emergency services arrive, the situation becomes more bearable.

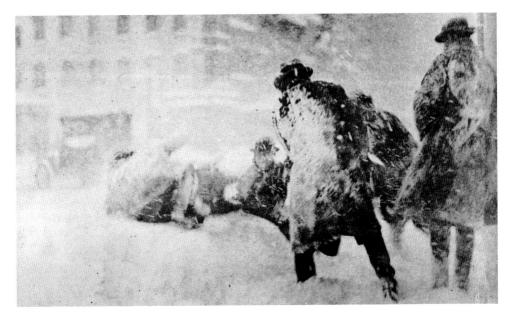

If you are outside and have metal objects with you, like an umbrella, or you are cycling, leave these in a safe place and continue your journey, since metal objects attract lightning. Do not go near telephone poles.

General advice

• When such storms occur, it is best not to go out at all, since during hurricanes or blizzards, there is minimal visibility, which increases the risk of falls and other accidents.

• Switch on the radio and follow the advice of the emergency services.

• All the family should keep away from electrical appliances in general, such as irons, computers, and televisions, etc. If possible, unplug all household appliances.

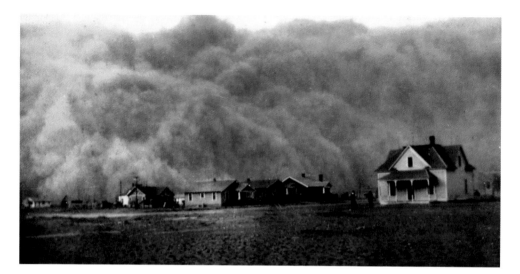

If a tornado takes you by surprise in the countryside, look for shelter in low places, such as hollows and ditches. It is best not to move from your shelter until the danger has passed.

• It is also advisable to keep away from doors and windows because of the risk of glass breaking, due to the force of the wind. A broken branch of a tree might be blown into the house and cause injuries to your family.

• Only use the telephone in case of emergency to avoid jamming the lines.

• If you have to go out into the street for any reason, cover yourself up well. Remember that mittens are warmer than gloves.

• When you are dressing, it is better for insulation if you wear several layers of thin clothing, rather than a single thick garment.

• If you encounter the storm while outside, try to take refuge in the doorway of a building or in low buildings. It is not advisable to approach trees or areas of high ground, because these are places at greater risk from a lightning strike.

• If you are outside, but in a car, try to stay inside it. Do not try to drive on flooded roads.

• If you are outside, but on a launch or sailboat with the sails up, try to reach port as soon as possible, or take down the sails, since they also attract lightning.

• If you are outside and feel tingling in your skin or your hair stands on end, lie down on the ground immediately because these are signs of an electric charge and you run the risk of being struck by lightning.

• Do not try to cross flowing water if the level is above your knees.

What to do if the storm is accompanied by floods

• When the storm is so intense that the natural riverbeds cannot contain the water, they overflow, causing a flood.

How to keep out of range of lightning?

• It is calculated that for an individual to be completely free from the effects of a lightning strike, he must be over 8 miles (13 km) from the origin of the bolt.

• To estimate the distance you are from where the lightning struck, count the seconds that elapse between the flash of lightning and the sound of the thunder. Divide the seconds by five, which will give you the distance in miles.

At times of heavy rain, keep away from the lowest areas in the house; go up to the higher floors, taking all your emergency supplies with you.

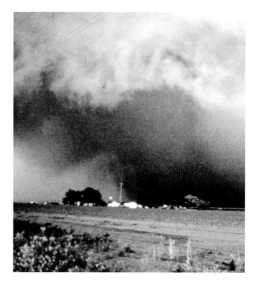

• When deciding where to live, find out where the water sources are. Do not build near riverbanks, since you run the risk of your home being flooded if they overflow.

• If your home is near places that habitually flood during the rainy season, get prepared for the situation. Phone the meteorological information service for the latest news when it rains heavily.

• Store enough drinking water for all the family to last a whole week, because during floods, pipes burst, which may interrupt the water supply. Also, store nonperishable foodstuffs, like canned food, dried fruit, or chocolate.

• Keep an emergency kit with your normal medication in a safe place in the house, enough for all the family for a week.

• Put a radio, a flashlight with spare batteries, and a camping stove in a safe place.

• You can also store tablets for water purification.

What to do after the flood

• Check all the household installations thoroughly: water, gas, and electricity. Call the insurance company to notify them of the damage caused by the storm.

• If, during the storm, some food has got wet from the rainwater, do not eat it, because you run the risk of getting an infection.

• Likewise, if the electrical appliances of the house have got wet, do not touch them and certainly do not switch them on.

• If there is no drinking water available after the storm, do not use water from wells or reservoirs, as they are very probably contaminated.

What should you do in the case of a tornado or hurricane?

• Seek refugee in buildings of solid construction. Avoid going near cabins or mobile homes. If the house has a basement, take refugee in it, as there you run less risk.

• Do not stay inside your car during a tornado or hurricane, because you run the risk of being dragged along by it.

• Avoid taking refuge in buildings with large roofs, such as sports centers, big tents, theaters or auditoriums, because of the risk of the roof coming off.

• If you stay inside your house, let down all the blinds and open one window on the opposite side to the wind. All members of the family should keep away from doors and windows.

Cold spells and heat waves

During periods when temperatures are extreme, you should take extra precautions. Elderly people and children should be given special supervision during these periods, in order to avoid any problems.

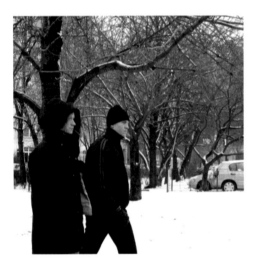

Cold spells

Periods of cold temperatures and snow, besides causing damage and giving rise to emergencies, cause increased susceptibility to viruses and bacteria, which affect mainly children and elderly people.

• If you live in an area that is often cut off by snow, work out how much food, water, and fuel are necessary for one week and store them in a safe place. Get hold of a camping gas stove.

• Add the medications that your family normally take to your household first aid kit.

• Make sure you have enough clothing in your closets to get through the cold spell.

• Check all the places where air gets into the house, such as doors and windows.

• Check your roofing and drainpipe system.

• Make sure your household heating system is not likely to freeze.

• Only use the telephone in case of emergency, so as not to jam the phone lines.

• Disconnect all electrical appliances that are not essential.

• Leave a faucet in your house trickling to prevent your water pipes freezing up.

• Do not in any situation allow children and elderly people to go out into the street, as they are the ones most sensitive to temperature changes.

Using your car during cold spells

• In a cold spell, only use the car if absolutely necessary.

• If you are going to travel by car, always take someone with you.

• Phone up the meteorological service to find out about weather conditions in the area you are going to drive through.

• Always take a fully charged cell phone when you travel.

• Before leaving home, fill the gas tank and do not wait until it is very low, before filling up again.

• Check the vehicle's antifreeze fluid, brakes, tire pressures, and spark plugs.

• The necessary items for a car journey during a cold spell are the following:

– Chains for the car to use in case of ice or snow.

– A shovel for removing snow.

– A flashlight with full batteries and spare batteries.

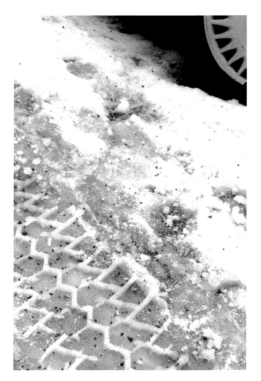

Drive very slowly in low gears, without following the tracks left by other cars. If you meet ice, try to head slowly toward areas of snow without braking at any time.

— High-energy foods, like chocolate or dried fruit.

• During the journey, tune in to radio broadcasts about the state of the traffic.

• It is not advisable to drive at night during snowstorms, because of increased risk of accidents.

• If the blizzard is so strong that you cannot continue the journey, stop your car and put the heater on. Leave one window slightly open to allow the air to be replaced and to avoid possible carbon monoxide poisoning. Put a conspicuous sign on the car's antenna to make it more visible.

• Get out of the car and check if it is covered in snow. If it is, remove it, taking care not to get burnt.

Heat waves

Heat waves have very negative effects, both social and economic. They are mainly a problem for the elderly, small children, and people with chronic illnesses, who have to take special precautions. In periods of very high temperatures, cases of fainting and dehydration increase and there is usually a higher incidence of allergies and insomnia than at other times of the year.

• Stay in the coolest areas of the house and seek out the shade as much as possible.

• If you are going to expose yourself to the sun, cover your head with a hat or cap and try to spend as little time in the sun as possible.

• Wear light transpirable clothing (clothing that "breathes") that is white or pale in color.

• Moisten your skin with towels soaked in cool water as often as possible.

• During the hours when the sun is strongest, lower the blinds and if you have sunshades, put them up.

• If you do not have air-conditioning in your house and the heat is too intense to bear, go to air-conditioned places, like shopping malls or cinemas, etc.

• The temperature of the air-conditioning should always be above 77°F (25°C).

• Do not play any sports during the sunniest period and reduce unnecessary physical effort wherever possible.

• Do not go out into the street during the hottest hours of the day.

• Avoid alcoholic drinks, coffee, or very sweet drinks.

• Do not take iced drinks, only very cool ones.

• Make light, cold meals, like salads and cold vegetables.

• Avoid eating food from mobile stalls, because their food goes off more quickly.

• If you are going to be in the sun, use high-factor sunblock.

• Always keep your hands clean.

In the car

• Your car should always have a good supply of water bottles, which are not kept in direct sunlight.

• When the air-conditioning is on, do not keep the windows completely closed, even if the car is in the shade or stopped.

• Use sun reflectors to prevent the car getting too hot.

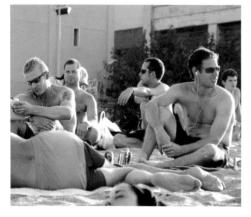

During heat waves, drink at least 4 pints (2 liters) of liquids a day, such as water, juices, and other refreshing drinks, even if you aren't thirsty.

Caring for the elderly and children

- Be very attentive to the nutrition and state of health of elderly people and children.

- Prevent children and the elderly being in direct sunlight; try to make sure they are always in the shade.

What to do if a person is suffering from heatstroke

- If a person has the following symptoms due to the heat, it is possible they are suffering from heatstroke:
    - Hot and red skin.
      Body temperature above 104°F (40°C).
    - Nausea and vomiting.
    - Convulsions and coma.

What should you do?

- Call the emergency medical services.
- Move the victim to a cool dry place.
- Lay him in a prone, supine position (lying on his back) with his head slightly elevated.
- Loosen the victim's clothing.
- Apply compresses soaked in cool water to his face and armpits.
- Give him cool water with a little salt to drink in little sips (1 teaspoon of salt per 2 pints (1 liter) of water.
- You can put him in a bathtub of cool water.
- If he is unconscious, do not give him liquids.

Avoid exercise in full sunshine during the hottest period.

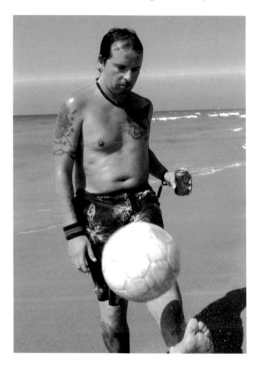

HOW TO DEAL WITH AN EMERGENCY

In accidents, first aid treatment can save people's lives

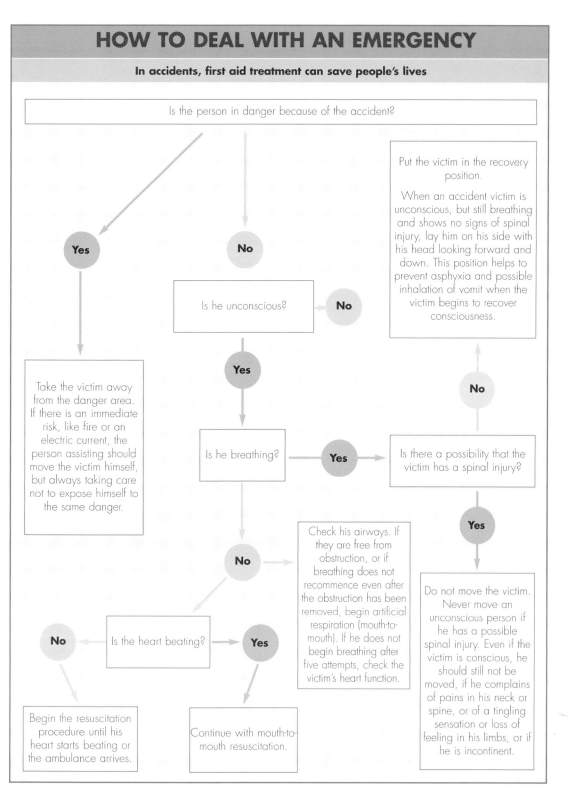

Is the person in danger because of the accident?

Yes

No

Put the victim in the recovery position.

When an accident victim is unconscious, but still breathing and shows no signs of spinal injury, lay him on his side with his head looking forward and down. This position helps to prevent asphyxia and possible inhalation of vomit when the victim begins to recover consciousness.

Is he unconscious?

No

Yes

Take the victim away from the danger area. If there is an immediate risk, like fire or an electric current, the person assisting should move the victim himself, but always taking care not to expose himself to the same danger.

No

Is he breathing?

Yes

Is there a possibility that the victim has a spinal injury?

Yes

No

Check his airways. If they are free from obstruction, or if breathing does not recommence even after the obstruction has been removed, begin artificial respiration (mouth-to-mouth). If he does not begin breathing after five attempts, check the victim's heart function.

No

Is the heart beating?

Yes

Do not move the victim. Never move an unconscious person if he has a possible spinal injury. Even if the victim is conscious, he should still not be moved, if he complains of pains in his neck or spine, or of a tingling sensation or loss of feeling in his limbs, or if he is incontinent.

Begin the resuscitation procedure until his heart starts beating or the ambulance arrives.

Continue with mouth-to-mouth resuscitation.

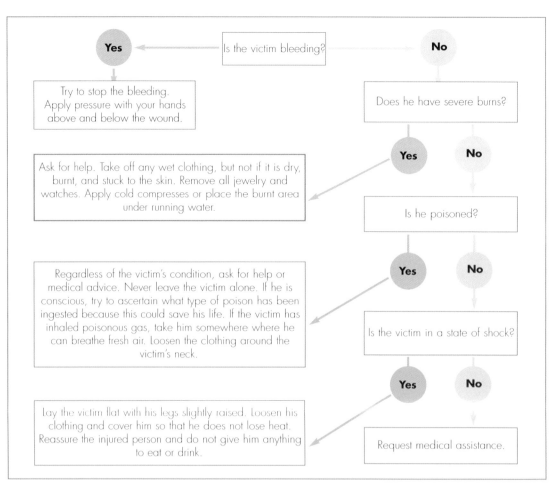

Yes — Is the victim bleeding? — **No**

Try to stop the bleeding. Apply pressure with your hands above and below the wound.

Does he have severe burns?

Yes   **No**

Ask for help. Take off any wet clothing, but not if it is dry, burnt, and stuck to the skin. Remove all jewelry and watches. Apply cold compresses or place the burnt area under running water.

Is he poisoned?

Yes   **No**

Regardless of the victim's condition, ask for help or medical advice. Never leave the victim alone. If he is conscious, try to ascertain what type of poison has been ingested because this could save his life. If the victim has inhaled poisonous gas, take him somewhere where he can breathe fresh air. Loosen the clothing around the victim's neck.

Is the victim in a state of shock?

Yes   **No**

Lay the victim flat with his legs slightly raised. Loosen his clothing and cover him so that he does not lose heat. Reassure the injured person and do not give him anything to eat or drink.

Request medical assistance.

◾ What should you check during an emergency?

- Is the victim breathing? If not, begin artificial respiration (mouth-to-mouth resuscitation) procedures.
- Is the victim's heart beating? If no pulse is detectable and you know how, begin the cardiopulmonary resuscitation technique.
- Is the victim unconscious? Place the person on his side with his head looking forward and slightly downward.
- Is there serious bleeding? If so, you must control it.
- Is the victim in a state of shock? If so, make him lie down with his feet up, cover him and reassure him.

◾ When should you call the ambulance or the doctor?

- Drowsiness for no apparent reason or loss of consciousness.
- Severe hemorrhaging.
- An unexplained fit of any kind.
- Breathing difficulties.
- Severe abdominal pain that does not stop after vomiting, which lasts more than three hours, and is accompanied by sweating and nausea.
- Blurred vision, seeing colored halos, or a sparkling aura around lights.